Arthritis of the Hip and Knee

About the Authors

Ronald J. Allen is the John Henry Wigmore Professor of Law at Northwestern University School of Law. He has written numerous books and articles on evidence and criminal procedure. He earned a J.D. from the University of Michigan. Both before and since his hip replacement operations, he has lectured all over Europe and in Australia and New Zealand.

Ron enjoys swimming, bicycling, and playing competitive tennis. Ron and his wife live in Chicago with their two daughters and two sons.

Dr. Victoria Anne Brander is Director of the Arthritis Center at the Rehabilitation Institute of Chicago (RIC), on RIC's Board of Directors, and Assistant Professor of Physical Medicine and Rehabilitation at Northwestern University School of Medicine. Vicky serves as President of the Illinois Society of Physical Medicine and Rehabilitation and as an advisor to the Women's Board of the Injury Prevention Program. She also serves on the Board of Directors of the Arthritis Foundation. She received her medical degree from Northwestern University Medical School and did her residency in physical medicine and rehabilitation at Northwestern University and RIC.

Vicky and her husband live in River Forest, Illinois, with their three young children.

Dr. S. David Stulberg is Professor of Orthopedic Surgery at Northwestern University School of Medicine and founder and director of the Joint Reconstruction and Implant Service at Northwestern Memorial Hospital. David earned his medical degree from the University of Michigan School of Medicine and served his residency in orthopedic surgery at the Harvard University Combined Orthopaedic Residency Program. He is a member of the Hip Society of America, a founding member of the Knee Society of America, a co-founder of the International Society for Technology in Arthroplasty, and a fellow of the American Academy of Orthopaedic Surgery. David is the author of numerous publications related to arthritis and joint reconstruction of the hip and knee, and he lectures frequently on these topics in America and abroad. He is a member of the Board of Directors at RIC.

David and his wife live in Chicago.

Arthritis of the Hip & Knee

The ACTIVE PERSON'S GUIDE to TAKING CHARGE

Ronald J. Allen
Northwestern University

Victoria Anne Brander, M.D.
S. David Stulberg, M.D.
Northwestern University
Northwestern Memorial Hospital
Rehabilitation Institute of Chicago

Patricia A. Lee
Contributing Editor

PEACHTREE
ATLANTA

Ω

Published by
PEACHTREE PUBLISHERS, LTD.
1700 Chattahoochee Avenue
Atlanta, Georgia 30318-2112

Manufactured in the United States of America

10 9 8 7 6 5

Library of Congress Cataloging-in-Publication Data

Allen, Ronald J. (Ronald Jay), 1948-
        Arthritis of the hip and knee: the active person's guide to taking charge /
by Ronald J. Allen, Victoria Anne Brander, S. David Stulberg . — 1st ed.
            p. cm.
        Includes index.
        ISBN 1-56145-149-5
        1. Total hip replacement—Popular works. 2. Total knee replacement—
Popular works.   I. Brander, Victoria Anne.   II. Stulberg, S. David   III. Title
RD549.A43   1997
617.5'810592—dc21

                                                                97-15388
                                                                CIP

Sixteen million persons in the United States suffer from osteoarthritis, the form of arthritis that is the focus of this book. If you have osteoarthritis in your hip or knee, you probably have seldom been encouraged to try to regain the active lifestyle you enjoyed before arthritis set in. If your experience is like that of most patients, young or elderly, you have been told that your only options for treatment are medications, minimal physical therapy, and, if needed, having your arthritic hip or knee replaced. You, your orthopedist, and your physical therapist may have all accepted that your being able to walk and to climb stairs is the reasonable extent of your physical abilities. Your expectations do not need to be so low. In this book, the traditionally held beliefs about the limitations of osteoarthritis treatment and the restricted roles patients play in their treatment are reevaluated.

This book shows that those of you who suffer from hip or knee arthritis should and can regain an active lifestyle. Taking control of your care—that is, (1) educating yourself about the disease, (2) becoming an active partner with your physician in the decision-making about your treatment, and (3) being determined and persistent in physical therapy—is the means to getting back the active, physically comfortable lifestyle that osteoarthritis took from you. The "Taking Charge" icons in the margins indicate text that details how you can actively participate in your treatment. Portions of the text that are called out in the margins highlight information that is especially important for you, the patient.

Arthritis of the Hip and Knee grew out of the experience of three persons who, through hard work and determination over many years, learned that the debilitating effects of osteoarthritis can be controlled. Ron Allen developed severe osteoarthritis of his hips at an early age and eventually had to have both of them surgically replaced. His first surgery, on his left hip, was in 1988. At that time, hip replacement was deemed successful if, following the surgery, the patient could walk without a limp and take part in the routine activities of daily living without great difficulty. The surgery was designed primarily to eliminate pain and not to restore a person to vigorous activity.

Ron found these limitations unacceptable. He had always lived a vigorous, athletic life and was unwilling to have his activity restricted so dramatically. He began on his own to press the then-accepted limits of rehabilitation, and two years follow-ing his surgery was able to play competitive tennis again. When his right hip had degenerated to the point where it, too, had to be replaced, Ron applied the lessons he had learned from his left hip. His right hip responded well to directed, systematic physical therapy, and within a few months Ron was back on the tennis court.

As Ron was working on his own to increase his level of activity, and thus the quality of his life, his surgeon, David Stulberg, was observing that many potentially very active pa-tients were also not achieving their full potential. This led David to conclude, as Ron already had, that the orthopedic community was systematically underselling the quality of life that patients with significant arthritis, as well as those with joint replacements, could achieve. David found a willing ally in Vicky Brander, a physician with a specialty in physical re-habilitation. David and Vicky began working together with patients of all ages who had osteoarthritis of the hip or knee, including Ron, and helped those patients achieve consider-able success in returning to an active life. David and Vicky found that anyone willing to make the effort to systematically apply a well-rounded arthritis program, with particular em-phasis on exercise, could accomplish what Ron had achieved.

Ron and David concluded that millions of people were liv-ing an impaired quality of life that, with knowledge and effort, could be dramatically improved. They decided to write a book, using Ron's case as an example, for individuals like you who have arthritis of the hip or knee, informing you how to make sure you get the best possible care, and the best possible re-sults. Because Vicky's participation was crucial both to the treat-ment of osteoarthritis and to the message of the book, she ea-gerly agreed to join the project. This book, then, is the result of the cooperative enterprise between an arthritis patient and his two primary doctors.

We hope that this book will encourage and inspire you to take charge of your osteoarthritis and to stay active.

Ronald J. Allen
Victoria A. Brander, M.D.
S. David Stulberg, M.D.

CONTENTS

Chapter 1
Introduction
1

Chapter 2
**Arthritis:
The Disease**
11

Chapter 3
**Living with
Arthritis**
27

Chapter 5
Preparing
for Surgery
105

Chapter 7
Post-Surgery
131

Chapter 8
Rehabilitation:
The Significance
of Physical
Conditioning
171

Chapter 9
Living with
an Implant
197

Chapter 10
The Future of
Care for Arthritis
of the Hip
and Knee
217

Arthritis of the Hip and Knee

INTRODUCTION

YOU MAY BE TWENTY, FORTY, sixty, or eighty years old, and you have things to do. You have always been active—mowed the lawn, played tennis, danced, shopped, just plain walked. Your health is fine, you have been active, and you definitely have the desire to stay active. But you can't because the pain in your hip or knee has become so severe that the things you like to do, the things important to you, are no longer fun and are starting to become difficult, maybe even impossible. You're not happy. And you're not alone. Millions of active people of all ages have hip and knee problems that are keeping them from doing the things they need and want to do.

Many people with chronic hip and knee problems have *osteoarthritis*, a disease that causes the progressive degeneration of a joint. If you have osteoarthritis, you may be unsure what to do. Should you try to tolerate the pain and hope it subsides? Should you see a doctor? You may be worried about the future. How quickly will the pain progress? Will you become even more crippled over time? How will this affect your life? How will it affect your family?

Like many people with osteoarthritis of the hip or knee, you have probably received conflicting answers to these and many other questions. You may be frustrated, depressed, frightened, or worst of all, immobilized. You're sure you do not have to endure this pain forever—or at least you hope you don't—but everything you have tried thus far has not worked to your satisfaction. You've reached the point where you are ready to take things into your own hands. We wrote this book on osteoarthritis to help you do just that.

 You can do many things to help rid yourself of that hip or knee pain so you can get back to the activities you need to carry out or wish to enjoy. Remarkable progress has been made since the 1970s in the medical, surgical, and rehabilitative treatment of arthritis of the hip and knee. The fact is that your chances are high of returning to anything you normally would be capable of doing if you did not have arthritis. The purpose of this book is to help you achieve that goal.

What You Need to Know

T O REACH YOUR GOAL of full, pain-free function, you need to know a number of things, and we provide them all in this book.

❑ *What is wrong with your hip or knee?* Chapter 2 explains how your hips and knees function and how osteoarthritis can cause you pain and decreased function in your joints.

❑ *How do you recognize and cope with the physical and emotional issues that result from arthritis?* Chapter 3 describes ways to manage your day-to-day activities and the various treatment options available, such as medications, exercise, and proper diet and nutrition.

❑ *What do nonsurgical and (if necessary) surgical treatments involve?* Building to the decision to undergo the most extensive treatment option, joint replacement surgery, is explained in detail for you. Although it is extremely unlikely that you will need such surgery, this information will help you understand your disease. Chapters 4–7 provide all the information you will need if you are considering or preparing for surgery (whether minor or major), from pre-operative planning to the surgery itself and through post-surgery recovery.

❏ *How large a role does exercise play in the successful treatment of hip and knee problems?* The role of exercise is enormous, and we reinforce this message throughout the book. But because its role is often misunderstood or undervalued, we devote Chapter 8 exclusively to this topic. The chapter stresses how to exercise appropriately and includes exercises for you to do at home.

❏ *If your arthritis warrants your undergoing a total joint replacement, how will you feel with the replacement inside your body?* What may be causing any pain you may be feeling? What happens should you reinjure yourself or require revision surgery? Chapter 9 answers these questions and more.

❏ *What treatment options are being developed?* To help you decide what course to follow now for your osteoarthritis, Chapter 10 looks at the future of hip and knee care and how to use new developments to your best advantage.

❏ *What have been some other persons' experiences with hip or knee replacement?* We outline below the experiences of Ron Allen, one of the authors of this book, with osteoarthritis of the hip, and he shares his thoughts in A Patient's Perspective sections throughout the book.

The more knowledge you gain about osteoarthritis, the more you will want to achieve the best results possible; and the more willing you are to work toward those optimal results, the greater your success will be. For this reason, the three of us—Ron Allen, a successful joint replacement surgery patient and a law professor; David Stulberg, an orthopedic surgeon; and Vicky Brander, a physiatrist (a physician who specializes in physical rehabilitation)—have collaborated to write this book. We wanted to provide insight into the thoughts and feelings of a team who together successfully cared for and treated a severe case of arthritis. Through our experiences, we hope you will be inspired to become an active participant in your own successful treatment.

A Patient's Experience

Ron Allen was thirty-four in 1982 when he learned that the pain he was having in his hips—pain that was interfering with many things he enjoyed doing, including playing competitive basketball and tennis—was the result of severe arthritis. Although he had been aware for some time that his legs did not feel normal, he was unaware that he had the disease, which most people associate with getting old.

In confronting his osteoarthritis, Ron initially sought to remain active without having to undergo surgery. Eventually, however, he realized that joint replacement surgery was inevitable for him, and as an active, young person he had to confront the implications of undergoing such surgery. Unwilling to compromise the level of his physical activity after surgery, Ron sought information that would allow him to continue living an active life. Ron had to tackle many of the difficult issues faced by active patients with serious hip or knee problems.

Considerations for Treatment

For six years, Ron sought ways to rid himself of his hip pain and maintain his active lifestyle. He had to learn about his disease and how to deal with it. How does an active young person confront the fact that he has a crippling disease of elderly people? How do persons of any age learn to handle the fact that their condition may gradually cause them to experience great pain and loss of function? Through well-constructed exercise formulated with the advice of experts in physical therapy and orthopedics, Ron's condition improved to the point where he had no symptoms for a time. But by 1988 Ron's left hip had deteriorated to the point where hip replacement surgery became necessary.

Now as a forty-year-old he was forced to learn about medical technology designed to relieve pain and restore normal joint function for seventy-year-olds! In the late 1980s, joint replacements were thought to last for ten years if you weren't overweight or very active, and if you were lucky. After that, the joint replacements could be redone, but second replacements were less durable than the original ones. Failure rates of revision procedures (which is the repeating of a previously done joint replacement) could reach twenty-five percent within three to five years. And what about third or fourth operations? Ron quickly calculated what he was facing, which was a life filled with major surgeries and increasing immobilization. Indeed, had Ron been sixty or seventy in 1988, as are most people contemplating joint replacement surgery, his life expectancy would have been fifteen to twenty years, and even then the odds of having a joint replacement last a lifetime wouldn't have been good! He probably would still need revision surgery in ten years. All of this was unacceptable to Ron, and he began a search for a better solution.

Was Ron able to get the information he needed to beat the odds he was facing? Yes. Can you? Absolutely! You not only can, but you *must* take an active role in preparing yourself, if treatment of your hip or knee is to be successful. We explain how in this book.

Surgical Considerations

DR. DAVID STULBERG KNEW THE prospects facing Ron. He knew how successful and durable joint replacement surgery could be in older, less active patients, but he was also very aware of how catastrophic it could be in younger, active patients. As an orthopedic surgeon, David specializes in joint replacement surgery, with a particular interest in joint surgery for young, active patients like Ron.

In the early 1980s, the technology of joint replacements

was in flux. By 1988, the surgical community had approximately twenty years of experience with *cemented* total hip replacements. In addition to his experience with cemented hip replacement, David had four years of experience with *uncemented* hip replacements. Ron spent many hours in the library researching the advantages and disadvantages of the options available to him. He and David had long discussions about the operation, the options, and the future. In 1988 Ron decided to have his left hip replaced and accepted David's recommendation to use a custom-made, uncemented artificial joint (prosthesis).

The surgery and immediate post-surgical recovery went extremely well; he was walking without support in six weeks. However, although his hip continued to improve over the next two years, he was not able to play active sports. Indeed, although Ron could engage in major life activities like walking and climbing stairs without pain, he was quite limited in what he could do.

Physical Therapy Considerations

MANY THINGS THAT MOST PEOPLE take for granted were difficult for Ron. Sitting for an extended period was uncomfortable. He could not easily bend down to pick up something, and using exercise equipment like a stair-stepper or treadmill was difficult. This situation was unacceptable to him. So each time he had difficulty moving in a certain way, he designed an exercise to work the relevant muscles, and each time the muscles responded. This led him to believe that he eventually could play tennis again. He set that as his goal, and he succeeded two years later.

During this time, Ron's right hip continued to deteriorate. During the winter of 1993, he had to give up playing tennis, and shortly thereafter, merely walking for more than fifteen minutes caused him intense, uncontrollable pain. It was time for the right hip to be replaced.

In 1993 at age forty-five Ron underwent the surgery on his right hip. Many things had changed in the five years since his left hip replacement. Orthopedic surgeons knew much more about uncemented hip fixation, and the new implants and surgical techniques reflected that additional experience. The rehabilitation program most suitable for Ron was not only understood by 1993, but was formalized under the direction of Dr. Vicky Brander, who specializes in physical rehabilitation.

The procedure and post-operative recovery went even better than expected—nothing short of amazing, in fact. Ron's progress can be attributed to several factors. Ron insists on being an active participant in decisions concerning his medical treatment, which is something not many patients do. In addition, he takes responsibility for his physical well-being, which contributes significantly to achieving positive results. For example, Ron began to strengthen the muscles of his right hip while it was mostly pain-free, so he would be physically prepared for the surgery when it came time. Also, the medical technology had improved.

Yet although his recovery was remarkable, Ron still had to accept that his hips were artificial and susceptible to all types of failure. In the years following his second replacement, he had to learn to live with his implants. For a while he did. Then in 1995 he fell in an ice-skating accident and fractured his left thigh bone (femur) near the first replacement. Now he had to deal with painful consequences that potentially could happen to anyone with a joint replacement. To complicate matters, signs appeared that indicated the plastic portion of his hip was beginning to wear and cause some of the bone to dissolve. He wondered, should he have the implant changed now or let the fracture try to heal? Would the fracture heal in the presence of worn plastic debris? If he waited to replace his hip, would there be enough bone left to attach a replacement? Had his tennis playing caused the plastic to wear? The accident generated deeper reflection on and an understanding of what it means to live with a total joint implant.

Ron was quite lucky. His fracture held in good position and the fixation of his hip implants was not disturbed. Yet the rehabilitation following the fracture was even tougher than it had been after his first total hip replacement. The pain lasted longer, and the strength and function of his hip took longer to return. Under Vicky's direction, new therapy programs were devised and carried out. By 1996, Ron returned once again to playing tennis.

Yet the fact that progressive bone loss was occurring because of continued wearing of the plastic was constantly present in his mind. When should something be done? he asked himself and David. Should he wait, as he had for his first replacements, until the pain was severe? Should the entire first left hip be replaced? How great were the chances for complications, like infection, with a second replacement? How long would the second replacement parts last? Would there be enough bone for a third replacement years later if it ever became necessary? All the potential risks were now real possibilities.

In the fall of 1996 Ron underwent a revision of his first hip replacement. The surgery and rehabilitation went more smoothly and quickly than he, David, and Vicky had dared hope. Ron is now walking better than he has since the 1970s and is also back playing active tennis.

Lessons Learned

ALL THREE OF US—Ron, David, and Vicky—have learned many lessons from Ron's more than fifteen years of physical therapy and three surgeries.

In the weeks after his first hip surgery, Ron learned two things: First, the medical profession doesn't listen to the needs of its patients as well as it should, and it underestimates patients' abilities to decide whether the care being prescribed for them is appropriate. Second, patients must actively enlist the cooperation of appropriately trained physicians and physical therapists to build a team that works together. Building a team can be frustrating and time-consuming, but it can ensure success. The willingness to participate in that process is a measure of a patient's desire to get well.

David learned lessons that physicians confronting frustrated, demanding patients must learn: that most failures of medical treatment are not the fault of the physician or of the patient. Rather, they result from physicians not actively encouraging patients to help themselves by taking some responsibility for their own care. Physicians bear a large portion of the responsibility for that encouragement.

Vicky has learned not to underestimate the patient's role in diagnosing and developing appropriate rehabilitation strategies. Many times, Ron complained of pain that sounded worrisome. She was able to help resolve this pain by modifying his aggressive exercise program. Vicky also learned that each patient handles confusing and difficult circumstances in different ways. For example, Ron needed to be intimately aware of every detail of his care and treatment and to be an active participant in decision making. Both she and David found that it was crucial to take the time to give Ron information—something doctors are finding less and less time to do these days.

Conclusion

Since 1988, Ron has had his left and right hips replaced, has fractured his left thigh, and has had to have his original left hip replacement redone. Today, Ron is pain free, playing active tennis again, teaching law, and with his wife raising a family of young children. Getting to this point has not been easy.

Ron knows he is living with artificial hips and that because he is young, a time may come when more treatment will be necessary. The details of Ron's experience are almost certainly different from what yours are and will be, just as the details of your orthopedist's care will almost certainly be different from David's, and the specifics of your physical therapy program will be different from Vicky's. Yet your feelings, and those of your surgeon and therapist, are likely to be similar to Ron's, David's, and Vicky's. The need to make decisions jointly as a team will certainly be the same. We hope that this book helps you to be an active participant in your treatment, to ask questions, receive answers, and make difficult decisions. Most importantly, we hope this book helps you achieve the kind of results that you have a right to expect.

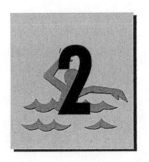

ARTHRITIS: The DISEASE

MILLIONS OF PEOPLE in the United States suffer from various joint problems. Many individuals are born with congenital abnormalities of their joints; others suffer injury from sports or accidents; still others develop problems as they age. More than one million persons have rheumatoid arthritis, a progressive inflammation and swelling of the joints. However, the most common joint problem, one that affects forty million Americans, is osteoarthritis, a progressive degeneration of the joints. It is this condition that is the main subject of this book. (See Table 2-1.)

Fortunately, medicine has made substantial advances since the 1970s in the treatment of joint problems of all types, including osteoarthritis. The progression of many of these conditions can be slowed. Effective treatment of the symptoms of joint problems (pain, swelling, and stiffness) is available. Daily activities, including sports, can often become possible, even for individuals with significant arthritis. Medical and rehabilitative interventions, if effectively administered

TABLE 2-1: The Socioeconomic Impact of Arthritis in the United States

Prevalence of Arthritis

❑ Arthritis is the number one cause of disability.
❑ More than 40 million persons show evidence of arthritis on x-ray.
❑ More than 16 million persons feel symptoms of arthritis.
❑ Up to 50 percent of persons 65 years of age and older have symptoms of joint pain, stiffness, or limitation of movement.

Costs of Arthritis

❑ Arthritis patients have more than 13 million doctor visits per year.
❑ Doctors prescribe over 12 million treatments or medications per year.
❑ Patients undergo more than 200,000 knee replacements each year.
❑ Patients undergo more than 150,000 hip replacements each year.
❑ Arthritis costs the economy more than $54 billion per year for medical care and lost wages or productivity.
❑ Sufferers spend more than $1 billion per year on unproven arthritis remedies.

Sources: Data from Arthritis Foundation, 1996 National Hospital Discharge Survey, Mercer Medical Cost Benefits Database; and from Commercial Assessment Document, *Osteoarthritis*, November 1994, Ciba.

and conscientiously accepted, can often postpone—and in some cases eliminate—the need for surgery, including joint replacements.

What Is Osteo-arthritis?

OSTEOARTHRITIS IS AN ABNORMAL CONDITION that causes a joint and its surrounding structures to deteriorate to varying degrees. (See Figures 2-1 and 2-2 on the stages of osteoarthritis of the hip and knee.) This degeneration in turn may cause pain and loss of function, also to varying degrees. One potentially frightening and occasionally harmful aspect of arthritis is that often its symptoms cannot be distinguished from normal physical sensations. Pain and stiffness, especially following vigorous activity, are often early symptoms of arthritis. They are also quite normal accompaniments of many

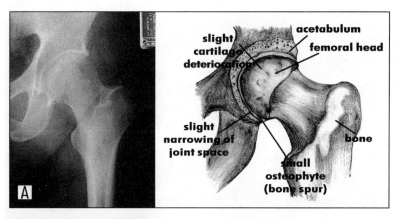

slight cartilage deterioration

acetabulum

femoral head

slight narrowing of joint space

bone

small osteophyte (bone spur)

A

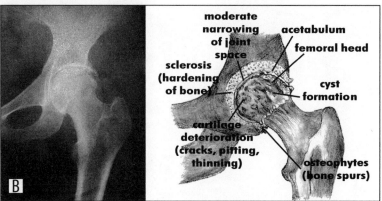

moderate narrowing of joint space

acetabulum

femoral head

sclerosis (hardening of bone)

cyst formation

cartilage deterioration (cracks, pitting, thinning)

osteophytes (bone spurs)

B

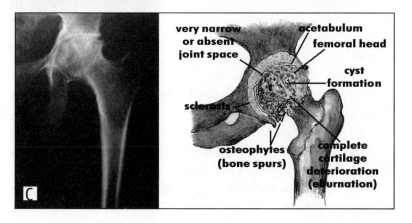

very narrow or absent joint space

acetabulum

femoral head

cyst formation

sclerosis

osteophytes (bone spurs)

complete cartilage deterioration (eburnation)

C

FIGURE 2-1
Stages of Osteoarthritis of the Hip

A. *Stage I: mild osteoarthritis*

B. *Stage II: moderate osteoarthritis*

C. *Stage III: severe osteoarthritis*

FIGURE 2-2
*Stages of
Osteoarthritis
of the Knee*

A. *Stage I: mild
osteoarthritis*

B. *Stage II: moderate
osteoarthritis*

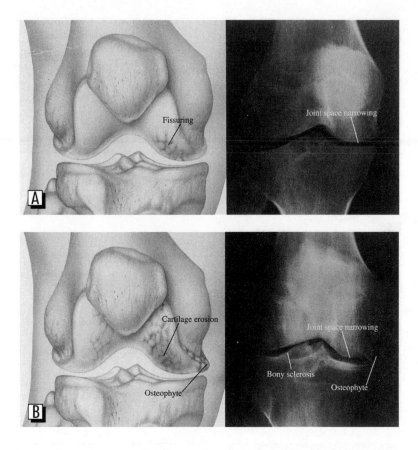

daily activities, especially those that exceed a person's level of conditioning.

If you are told you have arthritis, one of your first questions is likely to be, What caused this condition? Arthritis is a disease, not an aging process. Joints do not simply wear out. Many people grow old without ever developing arthritis; others develop arthritis in a few joints or just one joint. Many of the symptoms of aging, such as stiffness after sitting for long periods of time or soreness after walking long distances, are also symptoms of arthritis. However, merely having these symptoms does not necessarily mean you have arthritis.

Arthritis creates abnormalities within the structure of the joint. These abnormalities can cause the soft tissue that lines the joint (the synovium) to become inflamed, or they

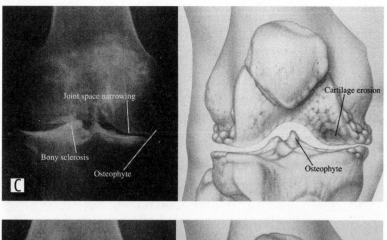

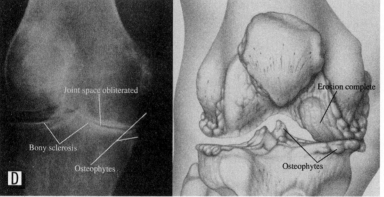

FIGURE 2-2

C. *Stage III: moderately severe osteoarthritis*

D. *Stage IV: severe osteoarthritis*

can cause the firm, smooth, shiny surface of the joint (the articular cartilage) to become thin and irregular. The bone under the cartilage may become very dense and stiff. Outgrowths, called osteophytes or spurs, may appear at the edge of the articular cartilage. These abnormalities within the joint cause weakness of the muscles and surrounding ligaments, joint instability, and pain.

Unfortunately, it is often not possible to determine what causes arthritis to develop in a particular joint. Some factors are known to have a role in the development of osteoarthritis; others are just suspect. Many of these factors follow.

❑ *Immune system:* Considerable recent study has focused on the role of the immune system in the development and progression of osteoarthritis. Although there is yet no practical, clinical application of these studies, this research may lead to some promising new drug therapies.

❏ *Early joint trauma:* Early joint trauma is known to lead to osteoarthritis, particularly if this trauma leads to injury to the bone, ligaments, or cartilage.

❏ *Joint stress, chronic injury:* Similarly, people who have jobs which require a significant amount of joint stress, and chronic repetitive injury (such as construction workers, football players) have significantly higher rates of osteoarthritis.

Recent research proposes a protective effect of exercise against the symptoms of arthritis.

❏ *Exercise:* Many investigators have looked for a link between exercise and the development of osteoarthritis. Several large, well-respected studies have found no increased risk for the development of arthritis in groups of athletes, such as long-distance runners. More recent research proposes a *protective* effect of exercise against the symptoms of arthritis.

❏ *Diet:* The role of diet in the development of osteoarthritis is unknown, although it also has been the subject of numerous studies investigating a potential relationship. Diets high in saturated fat, for example, have been theoretically implicated in the development of arthritis.

❏ *Genetics:* New insights into genetics have led to the discovery of inherited, familial forms of osteoarthritis associated with specific abnormalities of chromosomes.

Osteoarthritis is likely not one disease, but many. When the actual cause of osteoarthritis cannot be determined, the arthritis is called *primary*. If the cause of the arthritis can be determined, the arthritis is said to be *secondary*. As researchers identify the varying causes of osteoarthritis, more and more people are classified as having secondary arthritis. It is important to determine, whenever possible, the exact cause of arthritis so the condition can be treated appropriately. Sometimes the arthritis seen at the joint may just be an early or even initial clue to a more serious disease.

There are many causes of secondary arthritis of the hip and knee. For example, many fairly common childhood hip diseases, such as congenital hip disease, Perthes' disease, and slipped capital femoral epiphysis produce deformities of the hip joint that ultimately result in arthritis. Systemic diseases affecting metabolism, such as hemochromatosis and hypothyroidism, may cause identifiable forms of secondary arthritis. Other common causes of secondary arthritis are the disorders of crystal metabolism, such as gout and chondrocalcinosis. Blood disorders, such as sickle cell disease and thalassemia, are known causes of severe arthritis, particularly of the hips and knees. More rarely seen are the congenital abnormalities such as Ehlers-Danlos syndrome and hypermobility disorders, bone dysplasias, and other unusual familial syndromes. None of these conditions guarantees the development of arthritis. The rate at which arthritis develops when it occurs in these conditions varies greatly.

Other Forms of Arthritis

THE DISCUSSION THROUGHOUT THIS BOOK is dedicated to osteoarthritis. However, there are other, systemic forms of arthritis. Rheumatoid arthritis, systemic lupus erythematosis, and ankylosing spondylitis, among others, are diseases that cause different types of arthritis of the joints. These diseases, like osteoarthritis, cause pain and stiffness, but they also include a host of other medical conditions that do not occur in osteoarthritis. Like osteoarthritis, the treatment of these diseases requires exercise and the techniques of self-management that we describe in this book. Persons with these disorders frequently undergo joint replacement surgery. However, the overall approach to management, medication, exercise, timing of surgery, and other significant issues are different from osteoarthritis and so are not specifically addressed in this book.

How Is Osteo-arthritis Diagnosed?

THE FACT THAT ARTHRITIC SYMPTOMS are often non-specific and seemingly inconsequential explains, in part, why so many people with arthritis do not seek medical attention until their disease has progressed, often to a quite advanced stage. A delay in the diagnosis of arthritis not only causes what may be an unnecessary period of pain and loss of function, but may also affect the treatment options available. Although early symptoms of osteoarthritis can be partially hidden in the normal experiences of life, they can be identified if you or one of your acquaintances are even superficially knowledgeable about the disease.

Signs and Symptoms

PAIN AROUND THE HIP or knee may be due to many different conditions of the soft tissues, nerves, or bones surrounding the joint. Pain around the hip or knee may also be caused by a condition elsewhere in the body, such as in the back or abdomen. Hip arthritis is usually experienced as pain in the front and outside of the thigh extending into the groin. Knee arthritis typically causes an aching or gnawing pain directly at the knee that extends into the thigh or the lower leg. Pain is usually worsened by activities that involve bearing weight on the legs, such as walking or climbing stairs.

Early in the course of the disease, pain is rare. Stiffness goes away quickly when the affected joint is moved. Many people notice a cracking sensation of the joint, called crepitus. Although normal joints occasionally experience a cracking sound when, for example, a tendon passes over a bone, persistent cracking, especially if it is painful, may be due to arthritis.

Mild Arthritis

WHEN ARTHRITIS OF THE HIP or knee is mild, daily activities usually are not significantly compromised. For unknown reasons, the vast majority of people with arthritis remain at this mild level and their conditions do not worsen. If you have mild or even moderate non-progressive osteoarthritis, you can completely reverse your pain and disability with a properly applied medical and exercise program. We will show you how to do this in Chapter 8. If you have moderate or even fairly advanced non-progressive osteoarthritis and you continue your exercise program, you can ward off pain and stiffness for a surprisingly long time. Unfortunately, however, the disease does progress in many people.

Progression of the Disease

IF YOUR OSTEOARTHRITIS PROGRESSES, you will notice that you experience more intense pain and more noticeable stiffness. The pain and stiffness will occur more frequently during tasks that you once had been able to complete without pain. You will begin avoiding pain-inducing situations and movements. Instead of walking, you will take a cab. The speed of your walking will slow, perhaps dramatically. You may begin to limp. If your osteoarthritis progresses to an advanced stage, pain may become more constant, even awakening you at night. Your hip or knee motion will decrease. Sometimes, your joint may feel that it is going to give way with use. In general, you will find yourself becoming more sedentary.

Other Causes of Pain

HIP AND KNEE PAIN is frequently *not* caused by the arthritis seen on x-ray. A variety of conditions can cause discomfort of a joint: inflammation of the supporting structures, such as the bursae (causing bursitis) or tendons (causing tendonitis); fractures; pinched nerves in the back (causing radiculopathy or sciatica); or muscle sprains and strains. If you develop pain that does not go away after a few days of rest, you should see your doctor. Pain can be a danger signal, especially pain that is worsening or not abating quickly. A thorough physical examination and, if necessary, x-rays usually are all that are needed to discover the cause.

Physical Changes of the Hip

CHARACTERISTIC PHYSICAL CHANGES DEVELOP in people who have osteoarthritis of the hip and knee. If you have arthritis of the hip, you may notice that you are losing certain motions. The most typical types of decrease in motion are difficulty in spreading apart the legs (abduction), moving the leg straight back (extension), and turning the entire leg and foot inward (internal rotation). (See Figure 2-3.) Swelling within the hip joint, besides causing pain, makes it difficult to contract the gluteus medius, one of the muscles used in abduction of the hip. Ultimately, the swelling weakens that muscle and causes a characteristic limp. The limp is actually described as a lurch, an unconscious leaning over the impaired hip while walking. This leaning is the body's natural way of minimizing the weight placed on the hip.

Other conditions caused by the arthritis may contribute to a limp. The affected leg may be shorter than the unaffected leg, causing a limp and possibly even pain in the pelvis and lower back. The limp may also be caused by a shortening of the time that the foot of the affected hip actually touches the ground (shortened stance phase). Patients with an arthritic hip limp subconsciously to reduce painful weightbearing.

Physical Changes of the Knee

KNEE ARTHRITIS ALSO LEADS to characteristic physical changes, which cause pain and limit physical ability. Knee stiffness is common, especially in straightening out the knee (extension). (See Figure 2-4.) There may be a fixed bend (flexion contracture) of the knee. When the knee is bent, there may also be a secondary stiffness of the hip. The knee is more prone to swelling, which contributes to the feeling of tightness in or around the joint.

As a consequence of pain, immobility, and swelling, the muscles around the knee become weak, particularly the large muscles on the front of the thigh (the quadriceps). The thigh may become noticeably thinner. Long-standing arthritis of the knee can disrupt the surrounding ligaments, which may cause the knee to become unstable or to shift during movement. Sometimes the knee even develops an angular deformity, such as knock-knees or bowlegs. People with knock-knee or bowleg deformities often develop foot deformities; flat feet are particularly common. Knee arthritis causes the typical problems associated with walking, such as the development of a limp, reduced speed, and limited knee motion during walking.

Osteoarthritis can be easily identified, even in its early stages, by a knowledgeable physician who performs a careful

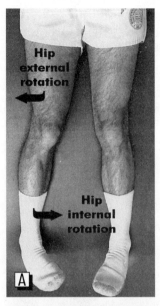
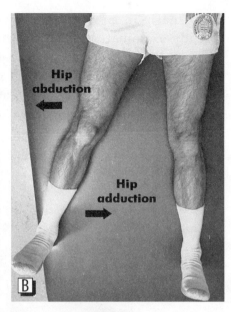
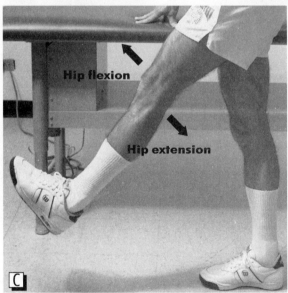

FIGURE 2-3
Motions of the Hip

A. *Hip external rotation (rotating straight leg so toes point to the outside) and internal rotation (rotating straight leg so toes point to the inside)*

B. *Hip abduction (moving leg out to the side) and adduction (moving leg back toward other leg)*

C. *Hip flexion (moving leg forward) and extension (moving leg backward)*

physical examination and takes routine x-rays. There are no specific laboratory abnormalities in persons with osteo-arthritis; laboratory studies are instead used to exclude other disorders when the diagnosis is not clear-cut. Occasionally, particularly in circumstances where the joint swells frequently, examination of the joint fluid may help sort out the cause of the arthritis. Remember, though, that simply having x-ray evidence of arthritis does not mean that the pain is a consequence of the joint degeneration seen on the x-ray. Numerous other conditions can cause pain, and many successful treatment strategies exist. The first step to feeling better is seeing a knowledgeable physician and obtaining an accurate diagnosis.

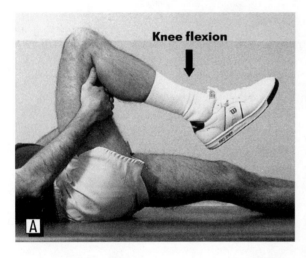

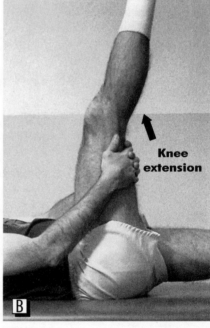

FIGURE 2-4
Motions of the Knee

A. *Knee flexion (bending knee)*

B. *Knee extension (straightening out knee)*

A Patient's Perspective: Ron

What Caused His Arthritis?

TWO THEORIES HAVE BEEN OFFERED to explain my arthritis. The first is that my hips were slightly deformed at birth—not enough to be noticeable by my family or my doctor, but enough to cause my hips to wear out at an early age. The second theory is that my arthritis resulted from a very bad break of my upper leg when I was fourteen years old and that caused my right leg to be an inch shorter than my left. I have learned that differences in leg length can result in unusual stress on the hips and pelvis, and possibly lead to faster than normal deterioration of the hip joints.

David doubts that the fracture of my femur led to the arthritis of my hips. He noticed very little deformity of my femur when he first examined me. Moreover, he said I developed arthritis of both hips almost simultaneously. He noted that I had no history to suggest I might have had a childhood hip disease, and also that if I had decreased my level of activity as a child and teen, when I had been very athletic, the lesser activity would not have prevented the subsequent deterioration of my hips.

In either case, my hips have been deteriorating for more than thirty years. Although it may seem odd, I had no idea that something was seriously wrong until the summer of 1982 when I saw an orthopedist and was diagnosed with severe osteoarthritis in both hips. Once the diagnosis was made, however, much about my personal health history came into focus, and a lot of things began to make sense.

What Took Him So Long to Seek Medical Care?

I FINALLY SAW A DOCTOR about my hips because, early in 1982, I had difficulty sprinting, even over very short distances. I first noticed this playing pickup basketball and did not think much about it. I attributed it to some passing ailment or being out of shape. Consequently, I spent some time trying to get in better shape, but for the first time in my life, my efforts paid no dividends. No matter what I did, I could not increase the flexibility in my legs, nor could I improve my foot speed.

During this time, I noticed a decline in my performance on the basketball court, soon followed by a decline on the tennis court.

I also began noticing greater pain and stiffness in my hips. On one occasion I remember walking up a flight of stairs and feeling a sharp pain in my left hip; on another, I had a similar pain bending down to pick up something. A number of people over these months had commented that I was limping, which I paid little attention to, because I did not really notice it myself, and I thought it to be just the result of too much strenuous activity. In the summer of 1982, I happened to walk past a storefront window and see my reflection. I saw for the first time what my friends had been commenting on. But I wasn't just limping; I was lurching. And I had been totally unaware of it.

My lack of self-awareness may seem odd, but in fact it is quite typical, especially of younger people with osteoarthritis. Because degenerative arthritis is often a slowly developing disease, my case had probably been developing since my mid-teenage years. As the disease developed, I naturally compensated for it without thinking. By the time I saw myself in the storefront window, I had probably been limping, first slightly and later much more dramatically, for years without knowing it as my body accommodated itself to the increasing stiffness and pain.

I now know that constant discomfort in the joints, even if it does not rise to the level of actual pain, is not natural and is an indication that something is wrong. If you can't move your leg without pain, or if you feel that something in the joint is blocking your progress, find out why. An example, which at the time I completely ignored, occurred when I was in college, over a decade before I was diagnosed with arthritis: I could not lean back comfortably in a car. Why not? Because when you lean back in a car, your pelvis and hips move forward over the car seat, freeing up your legs to swing outward and allowing your knees to separate. Whenever I did that, I could not get comfortable, because as my knees parted, my hips hurt. I had to prop my legs against something, like the side of the car. Why didn't I realize something was wrong? This discomfort was quite natural for me, and I always had an excuse, such as overdoing it on the basketball court or skiing recently.

As MY EXAMPLE OF EXPERIENCING PAIN while leaning back in a car suggests, the very best clue that something might be wrong is when you cannot do easily and painlessly the normal day-to-day tasks that others can do. Getting into and out of cars actually involves considerable flexibility. If you find it difficult to get in or out, something is probably wrong. Going up and down stairs should be easy and fluid, but often it is not so for people with arthritis. If you get stiff simply sitting for a moderate length of time or if you cannot cross your legs easily or sit on the ground comfortably, something is wrong. Normal everyday acts should not be difficult or painful, *but if they are, look into it!*

It is especially important for the highly active person to know that the saying "no pain, no gain" is false. Ironically, from age fourteen to about age thirty-five, I actually believed it was true because every time I worked out strenuously, I hurt badly. Such pain is not natural, especially if the pain and stiffness are in the joints rather than the muscles. This is not always easy to distinguish, mainly because very few people think of the distinction. Pain in the muscles can be benign, but pain and stiffness in the joints need further investigation.

Do not be misled by the fact that although you may feel stiff, you will soon loosen up. For years, as my arthritis got worse, I could force my body to loosen up sufficiently to play full-court basketball and very high-level tennis. My tennis partners often joked about how I would limp onto the court obviously looking for sympathy and then play as though nothing was wrong. Well, something was very wrong, but in those limited circumstances and for a short period of time, I was able to overcome it. Having to overcome pain such as this is yet another sign that something may be wrong.

Another early sign that often occurs is the feeling that one of your joints is filled with corn flakes when you first get up in the morning or first begin more strenuous activity. I remember many years ago feeling a slight crunching sensation that would go away almost immediately upon walking, but as time passed it persisted longer and longer. Joints should not crunch, at least not consistently; *but if they do, look into it.*

What Advice Does He Give for Seeking Care?

Conclusion

B Y BECOMING KNOWLEDGEABLE about your condition, you can make better choices about how to treat it. If you have early stages of arthritis, it is possible to slow the progress of the disease or at least to dramatically extend the time the joint takes to disintegrate. In addition, strengthening and flexibility regimens can greatly reduce discomfort and increase performance, even for those who do not wish to otherwise modify their activities. Knowledge is power, so keep your eyes open and listen to your body. It may be trying to tell you something important.

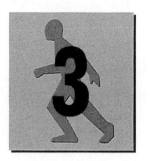# LIVING with ARTHRITIS

RTHRITIS, LIKE ALL CHRONIC DISEASES, does not go away. Its symptoms may be controlled, even eliminated. Its impact on your life may be greatly reduced. But its presence, even if removed surgically, is potentially always there. This idea can be terrifying and depressing. What does it mean to have a disease that conjures up ideas of an inexorable increase in pain and loss of function? Should you change your life? Can you travel, or play sports, or kneel in the garden? Must you consider yourself ill? The specter of arthritis can affect every aspect of your life. Yet millions of people with arthritis of the hip and knee live full, normal lives. How have these people done it? The same way you can and will do it. First, however, it helps to know what it is like to live with arthritis. That is the purpose of this chapter.

Take Control of Your Life

LIVING WITH ARTHRITIS affects you both physically and emotionally. You have daily responsibilities and activities, so how do you function effectively and efficiently? This is the physical issue. You also have to interact with your friends, family, business associates, and others. Even interacting with close family and friends can become complicated; you want to enjoy life and normal activities but become frustrated by your limitations, which regrettably you may take out on the people you are closest to. You may find yourself feeling depressed. These are the emotional issues associated with living with arthritis.

The physical and emotional issues of living with arthritis are distinct but intimately related. The best solution to the physical limitations caused by arthritis is to reduce the difference between the world of arthritis and the healthy world as much as possible. Doing so has tremendous emotional benefits. Reducing the distance between the worlds requires you to take control of your life in many ways, which we describe in this chapter. Taking control of your life often drastically changes your outlook from that of a victim to that of one in control who is maximizing his or her potential. If you combine that change with intelligent regulation and modification of your environment, your life will become considerably more enjoyable. Because the emotional issues of living with arthritis influence the way you deal with the physical issues, we address those physical issues first.

Overcome the Physical Issues of Arthritis

PHYSICAL ISSUES OF ARTHRITIS INCLUDE general mobility, which you can greatly improve by exercise, and your cherished activities, which you may need to adjust some but should not stop doing.

THE MOST IMPORTANT FACTOR that will improve the quality of your life is overall physical conditioning. The second most important factor is developing strength and flexibility in your affected joint. The discomfort of arthritis is much easier to bear if the rest of your body is in good shape. Being in good overall physical condition makes everything else easier. It's hard enough walking up stairs with a sore hip. It's all the more difficult if you are huffing and puffing by the time you have gone up halfway. So keep yourself in good physical condition through sensible physical activity that helps build and maintain both general strength and aerobic conditioning.

Aerobic exercise, which is important for all of us, is particularly critical if you have arthritis. Persons who have arthritis and tend to be sedentary have significantly reduced heart and lung capacity compared to others their own age who do not have arthritis. This can be reversed with regular aerobic exercise. By far the best aerobic activities for those with arthritis in the hips and knees are swimming, cycling, and if tolerable, walking. None of these activities will increase the rate at which your joint deteriorates. In fact, medical studies have been unable to find any connection between even considerable amounts of exercise, including running, and the development or progression of osteoarthritis of the hip or knee. Aerobic exercise also helps keep your weight under control, which will help reduce the symptoms of your arthritis and will make you feel better about yourself.

Restoring strength and flexibility to the arthritic joints is the second important component in improving the overall quality of your life. The pain and stiffness associated with arthritis are caused two ways. The first is the breakdown of the joint itself, and the second is the weakening and tightening of the muscles and soft tissue structures surrounding the joint. As your joint deteriorates, you will tend to use it less by reducing your activity. Joint cartilage needs motion and stress to repair itself and remain healthy. An immobile joint deteriorates faster. Immobility also causes the muscles around the affected joint to weaken. Weak muscles cannot function well

Exercise, Exercise, Exercise

The best aerobic activities for those with arthritis in the hips and knees are swimming, cycling, and walking.

as efficient shock absorbers for the joint and, therefore, are less effective in protecting a joint from pain and deterioration. Thus, strength and flexibility exercises are essential to reduce pain and to slow or reverse the progression of arthritis.

Don't Stop Doing What You Love

UNFORTUNATELY, ARTHRITIS OF THE HIP and knee can make cherished activities, including sports, difficult. Whether the activity is gardening, golf, or tennis, you may feel that you must choose between continuing your hobby or suffering more because of it. The suffering may be physical, such as stiff joints the day after a tennis match, or emotional, from having to witness what you consider your limited performance. Giving up your sport or hobby means giving in to arthritis. And giving in leads to self-pity and depression. Instead, accept performance that is not perfect and learn to modify what you want to do so you can continue to do it.

Learn and respond to your limits for activities that require you to be more physically active. If, for instance, you love to play golf but have difficulty getting into and out of a golf cart, then sit more on the edge of the seat with your afflicted leg resting on the outside edge of the cart, rather than bringing it all the way into the cart.

Periodically Loosen Up

MOST INDIVIDUALS WITH ARTHRITIS REPORT that they have difficulty arising from chairs and feel persistent stiffness and pain after sitting for prolonged periods of time. The best way to limit the discomfort is to make sure that you stand up and walk around to loosen up every thirty to forty-five minutes. If certain kinds of chairs lead to discomfort, don't sit in those chairs. Soft, low chairs without arms are very difficult to rise from. Instead, sit in a high surface chair with arms.

Sitting in one position for long periods of time (such as in a car or an airplane) can actually trigger a serious flare-up of arthritis pain. Limit periods of driving so you can stop and stretch, and make sure that you ask for aisle seats on a plane or train.

In Chapter 8, we discuss exercises that properly build

and strengthen the hips and knees. Doing these exercises will increase the quality of your life, reduce pain and disability, and help you delay or avoid surgery. But we also encourage you to see a physical therapist or a physiatrist for an exercise program. These specialists will be able to help you tailor a workout regimen to your special needs.

I N 1982, WHEN I WAS DIAGNOSED with severe arthritis, I was in serious pain, and my left hip was essentially immobile. I walked with a very bad limp and could not straighten my left leg. I began a therapy regimen designed to build up strength and flexibility in the hip, and within two months I was close to being asymptomatic. I had almost no pain and was walking without a limp. I did give up basketball, which was the sensible thing for me to do, but I was able to continue playing tennis actively. This lasted through 1988, by which time my left hip had deteriorated to the point that surgery was inevitable. The lesson here is that intelligent exercise transformed me for a six-year period, greatly increasing the quality of my life and postponing surgery for a number of years.

A Patient's Perspective: Ron

A RTHRITIS CAN MAKE virtually any movement or daily activity more difficult. Dressing, getting in and out of cars or chairs, going up stairs, and using the bathroom can all be impeded by stiff and sore joints. Arthritis can even disturb sleep. In dealing with arthritis-induced impediments to daily life, keep in mind that you can modify what tasks you do and alter your environment in innumerable ways to make your life less difficult. (See Table 3-1 for principles of joint protection.)

Make Your Daily Activities Easier

YOU CAN EASILY MODIFY your daily hygiene activities to accommodate your arthritis. Many tools are available to help you accomplish this, so ask your physician or an occupational therapist for information about local medical supply companies or mail-order catalogs.

Personal Hygiene

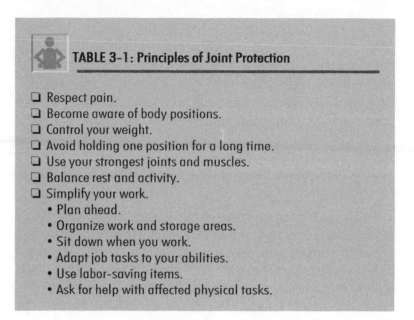

TABLE 3-1: Principles of Joint Protection

❏ Respect pain.
❏ Become aware of body positions.
❏ Control your weight.
❏ Avoid holding one position for a long time.
❏ Use your strongest joints and muscles.
❏ Balance rest and activity.
❏ Simplify your work.
  • Plan ahead.
  • Organize work and storage areas.
  • Sit down when you work.
  • Adapt job tasks to your abilities.
  • Use labor-saving items.
  • Ask for help with affected physical tasks.

Bathing

Bathing can be a difficult activity if you have arthritis. A walk-in shower is easier to use than a bathtub, which requires you to step up to get in and out of it. Reaching down to wash your feet can be a problem, so use a long-handled sponge, which is readily available. If you only have a tub to bathe in, you should purchase one of the many types of bath benches that are available; some benches simply sit inside the tub like a chair, whereas others swing out and back into the tub to make transfers easier. (See Figure 3-1.) If you use a bath bench, you may wish to install a hand-held showerhead and, if needed, a handrail on the wall or tub to help you rise safely from the tub. This may sound like a lot of equipment, but you can obtain and install these devices easily.

Going to the Bathroom

Elevated toilet seats are an easy solution to the problem of frustratingly low toilet seats present in most homes. Elevated toilet seats are available in many types, from simple foam cushions and inexpensive plastic donuts to more sophisticated adjustable seats. Some raised seats come with handrails attached. Or you can purchase handrails separately

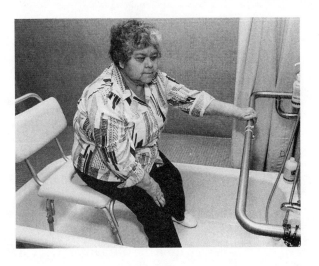

FIGURE 3-1
Bath Bench

and install them easily on the toilet for added stability and assistance. (See Figure 3-2.)

WHEN SIMPLE ACTIVITIES of daily living, such as dressing (especially your lower body), become difficult to perform—even though you are exercising and stretching regularly and you have modified your environment or your technique—you may wish to consult an occupational therapist. The occupational

Dressing

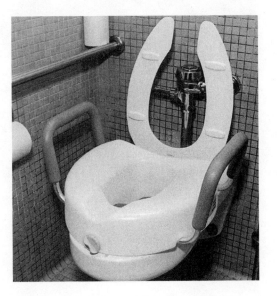

FIGURE 3-2
Raised Toilet Seat with Rail

therapist will evaluate how you perform an activity, offer suggestions on different ways to perform the task, and help you decide if a specific tool or aid can assist you in performing the activity more easily.

Being open-minded about using a self-help device is the key to success. Some people feel that using adaptive equipment is obtrusive and unattractive—the equipment reminds them of their disabilities. We suggest, however, that rather than viewing these devices as a sign of weakness, you consider them instead as technology that helps you perform tasks more easily, much as a power mower makes mowing the lawn easier.

You can overcome the difficulties with lower body dressing by using some very simple equipment. When arthritis limits your motion at the hip or knee, bending to the floor or reaching your feet is nearly impossible. Long-handled equipment overcomes this impairment. Sock donners help you put on socks, extended handle shoe horns assist with shoes, dressing sticks facilitate pulling up pants, and reachers pick up items off the floor. (See Figures 3-3 to 3-5.)

FIGURE 3-3
Sock Donner

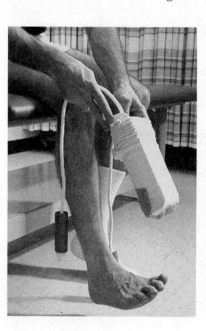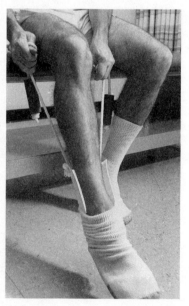

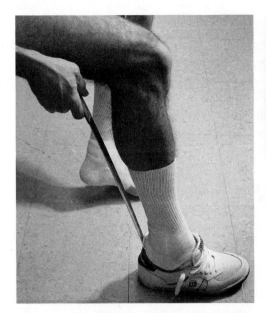

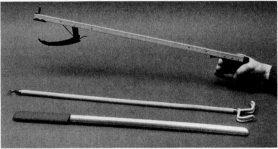

left,
FIGURE 3-4
Extended Handle
Shoe Horn

above,
FIGURE 3-5
Dressing Sticks
and Reacher

D RESSING CAN BE A GREAT PAIN, literally and figuratively, for someone with arthritis of the hips and knees. Putting on socks and shoes in the conventional manner became very difficult for me (socks, in fact, became impossible for a while) because of my declining flexibility, as did putting on underwear and pants. But you don't have to dress yourself in the conventional manner; you can change both your environment and the way you interact with it.

Slip-on shoes like loafers, for example, can replace shoes that tie and allow you to avoid the pain and frustration of trying to tie your shoes. You don't always have to wear socks, especially with slip-on shoes, and if you have to wear socks, a very inexpensive device is available to help you put them on. If you have to wear shoes that tie, you don't have to bend down to tie them while your foot rests on the floor. You can put your foot up on a step to tie it, or, as I did, simply put one foot on top of the other. That much additional elevation turned an impossible task into a simple one for me. And do not hesitate to ask your family or friends for help. I can assure you that they will be glad to be called on and will not view it as a burden. With pants, you don't have to stand and put

A Patient's Perspective: Ron

one leg in at a time. You can sit on the edge of a bed or chair and easily slip them on.

The Importance of Proper Footwear

Many people with arthritis of the hip or knee develop flat feet and have pain in their ankles and feet. Proper footwear can reduce hip and knee pain as well as ankle and foot pain. If you have fairly normal feet, you should wear shoes that are wide and deep, with firm arch supports and low, wide heels. (See Table 3-2.) If you have deformities, or arthritis in your feet, you may need orthotics or special shoes. An orthotist may be very helpful in assessing your needs.

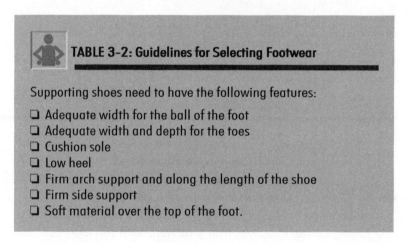

TABLE 3-2: Guidelines for Selecting Footwear

Supporting shoes need to have the following features:

- ❑ Adequate width for the ball of the foot
- ❑ Adequate width and depth for the toes
- ❑ Cushion sole
- ❑ Low heel
- ❑ Firm arch support and along the length of the shoe
- ❑ Firm side support
- ❑ Soft material over the top of the foot.

Other Useful Adaptive Devices and Equipment

Many medical supply companies in the United States offer adaptive equipment that can make daily life easier for you. Ingenuity and innovation by individuals with impairments have greatly improved the quality and number of aids available commercially. For example, there are special stools to help gardeners work more efficiently without hurting their joints, special handles to help open jars for people with arthritic hands, and a host of other practical equipment. If you wish to rent or purchase adaptive equipment, consult your physician or an occupational therapist to assist you in identifying the equipment best suited for your needs.

Alternatively, the Arthritis Foundation produces a number of comprehensive catalogs of adaptive equipment designed for people with arthritis. Their regular reviews of equipment, as well as new medications and treatment strategies, are an invaluable source of up-to-date information. To contact the Arthritis Foundation, receive the equipment catalogs, or subscribe to its journal, call 1-800-933-0032.

Common Activities in the Home and Workplace

EVERYDAY ACTIVITIES, SUCH AS WALKING, climbing stairs, getting in and out of chairs and cars, and simply trying to complete chores or work tasks can provide major obstacles if you have arthritis of the hip or knee.

Using a Cane

Most people tolerate severe joint pain and weakness before using an assistive device, such as a cane, for walking. However, a cane—placed in the *opposite* hand if there is hip arthritis or the hand on the *same side* for knee arthritis—can help you walk comfortably and for longer distances. Once you begin to walk with a limp on a regular basis, it is time to start using a cane. It is much better for you to walk normally and for long distances with a cane than abnormally and for short distances without a device.

Climbing Stairs

Climbing stairs is one of the most difficult activities for persons with an arthritic hip or knee. The first solution is to avoid stairs if you can. A better solution is simply to take your time, and always use the handrail. On days when you are in serious pain, walk up one step at a time, leading *up with the good leg* and *down with the bad leg*. If you must climb stairs and there are no handrails, it may help to use a cane.

Getting In and Out of Chairs

Low-slung, soft chairs and sofas are the most difficult for persons with arthritis to get out of. Don't sit in them. The lower the seat of the chair, the more difficult it will be for you to arise. Try to always sit in the highest chair in the room. Also, the lower the height of the chair, the more you will need your arms to push yourself up. Look for chairs with arm rests. This will vastly improve the ease with which you get up and out of the chair.

If it becomes difficult to arise from standard height chairs with arm rests, you still have options available for your home or workplace. First, try placing a large firm cushion or telephone book on the seat of the chair to raise the height of the seat. Spring-loaded cushions are commercially available that provide an additional boost as you get up from a chair. There are also electric chairs in which the seat raises and tilts to help you out of a chair. However, these are probably no more effective—and quite a bit more expensive—than simply raising the height of a seat with a very firm cushion.

Getting In and Out of Cars

When getting in and out of cars, make sure that the seat is positioned to give you maximum room. Take your time and move slowly. Much of the frustration and discomfort with everyday activities comes from trying to do them as quickly as you had been able to. Just accept the fact that for you time has slowed down somewhat, and don't worry about it. It takes a normal person about two seconds to get into a car. If it takes you five seconds, you will not have disrupted anybody's schedule.

Work at Home and in the Office

Arthritis of the hips and knees can cause problems while working—whether that work is homemaking, childrearing, in an office, or out of doors. The difficulty climbing stairs, bending, and carrying heavy objects can make housekeeping dreadful. Standing at the sink cleaning dishes becomes painful. Carrying children up stairs can become impossible. Prolonged sitting at a desk or in a meeting can cause considerable stiffness. When you finally arise, your stiffness may be painful and embarrassing. Work that requires long periods of standing, walking, and carrying heavy objects may become very difficult. Construction jobs may become impossible to perform.

The first step in dealing with these difficulties is to analyze them carefully. Break tasks down into smaller components, and use the joint protection principles and energy conservation techniques that we provide in this chapter. (See Tables 3-1 and 3-3.)

At home, for example, don't run up and down the stairs twenty times a day. Accumulate items on the steps and carry them all up at once—or get someone else to carry them up at the end of the day. Stand at the sink with your arthritic leg on a step stool; you'll be surprised how this helps relieve back and leg pain.

At work, modify your workspace to accommodate your physical needs. Change your chair or the height of your desk.

If you are still having trouble at home or at work, then get a referral from your doctor to see an occupational therapist. If your employment situation is becoming intolerable because of the arthritis, consult a vocational rehabilitation counselor. These individuals are trained to work with employees and employers to accommodate worker's needs. Since the passage of the Americans with Disabilities Act, employers are obliged by law to make reasonable accommodations for workers' physical needs.

F ATIGUE IS A VERY DISABLING ASPECT of arthritis. And it *does* take more energy to live with arthritis. Fatigue may come as a consequence of poor sleep; it may be a manifestation of a growing emotional weariness of the continued struggle against pain and disability; or it may occur simply from the boredom of your increasingly sedentary life. Depression and anxiety certainly intensify fatigue, and so does a lack of exercise. In addition, many medications used to treat arthritis and its pain can cause fatigue as a side effect.

Get Enough Rest

Increasing your physical activity will improve your body's endurance for daily activities and reduce the fatigue you experience in the late afternoon and early evening. Learning and applying techniques of energy conservation can be helpful. (See Table 3-3.) Perhaps most important is developing the mindset that fatigue is a challenge to be conquered, so that you don't let it depress you.

A Patient's Perspective: Ron

I HAD THE DISTINCT IMPRESSION, whether scientifically accurate or not, that I was expending an enormous amount of energy dealing with the symptoms of arthritis. As everything becomes more difficult, more energy is required to do anything. In addition, I had the sense that merely coping with the pain was draining. In fact, I believe that in each of the years leading up to my surgeries I suffered considerably more from colds and infections than at any other time of my life, and I attribute this to the increasingly debilitating pain I suffered. Adequate rest thus becomes doubly important, but with a grim irony, arthritis can interfere with your sleep. Thankfully, there is much you can do to combat this particularly frustrating consequence of arthritis.

TABLE 3-3: Energy Conservation Techniques

❑ Use proper body positioning during rest and activity. Poor body mechanics, such as stooped shoulders or too low a table height at work, increases the energy spent.
❑ Take breaks.
❑ Pace your activities.
❑ Prioritize. On days when your arthritis is painful, do only critical errands and save the routine chores for when you feel better. Let others do tasks that need to be accomplished but can be performed by someone other than you.
❑ Plan ahead to conserve steps. Store items on the stairs throughout the day and then carry them upstairs at one time.
❑ Simplify jobs.
❑ Use adaptive equipment.
❑ Sit on a stool instead of standing when you prepare dinner.

Note: *Rehabilitation through Learning: Energy Conservation and Joint Protection Techniques* by G. P. Furst explains these techniques in detail. It is available at your library, your local chapter of the Arthritis Foundation, or the U.S. Department of Health and Human Services.

Sleeping

IT IS CRITICAL THAT YOU IMPROVE the quality of your sleep. Most people sleep about seven or eight hours per night, but as we age, we begin to experience a decline in both the quality and duration of our sleep. Good sleep habits can maximize your chances of getting a good night's sleep. Table 3-4 lists some things you can do to help ensure sound sleep.

Even if you regularly practice good sleeping habits, arthritis can and will intrude upon your sleep. Pain fragments sleep, causing you to awaken many times during the night and to have light, easily disrupted sleep. This kind of sleep is much less efficient and causes many people with arthritis to become fatigued.

Find a Comfortable Position

One particularly troublesome byproduct of arthritis during sleep is that it becomes increasingly difficult to straighten your leg in relation to your body, especially at night. You cannot lie on your back or your stomach comfortably. When you lie on your back, your leg hurts unless you bend your knee. When you lie on your stomach, the hip or knee joint is being stretched, which also hurts.

Sleeping on your side avoids this problem. However, it may be possible, by stretching the muscles along the front of your lower body (the hip flexors and knee extensors), to continue to sleep comfortably on your back or stomach. To stretch these muscles, lie on your stomach on a flat, firm surface, just as though you were in bed trying to sleep in this position. Keep your legs straight, and you will immediately feel the muscles stretching out. If you can't lie flat in this position, then bend slightly at the waist, but be sure to keep your heels pointed straight toward the ceiling. Lie in this position for no more than a couple of minutes (less if it hurts too much), and you will feel your muscles begin to stretch.

Do this every day, and you will soon notice that, as the thigh muscles are stretching out, it becomes increasingly comfortable to lie on either your stomach or your back. You will also notice that it becomes more comfortable to walk. Performing this simple stretching exercise may return enormous benefits in comfort.

TABLE 3-4: Proper Sleep Habits

❑ Develop regular sleep patterns.
 • Go to bed and arise at the same times each day, even on weekends.
 • Avoid daytime naps.
 • Take a hot bath or drink a hot beverage (such as milk or noncaffeinated tea) before bed.
 • Establish a bedtime ritual.

❑ Optimize your sleep environment.
 • Don't eat large meals within two to three hours of bedtime.
 • Make sure your sleeping environment is dark, quiet, and comfortable.
 • Keep the clock face turned away from you.

❑ Exercise.
 • Exercise regularly, both aerobically and for strength and flexibility, to maximize physical comfort during sleep.
 • Don't exercise immediately before bedtime.

❑ Avoid drugs that interfere with sleep.
 • Don't smoke. If you do smoke, don't smoke before bed.
 • Limit alcohol to one to two drinks per day at most.
 • Eliminate caffeine from your diet.

❑ Reduce stress and anxiety.
 • Use stress-reduction techniques such as meditating, listening to music, and stretching each day.
 • Before bedtime, collect your thoughts and write down a list of tasks you need to accomplish the next day so your sleep won't be disturbed by worries.

Another common problem at night is that your leg hurts when it rotates. If you are lying on a flat surface with your toes pointing toward the ceiling, your legs typically will rotate away from your midline when you relax your muscles. As your joint gets worse, this can be painful as bone rubs on bone. Little in the way of exercise can help this, but a pillow might. Resting your leg on a pillow gives it rotational support as it settles into the pillow, thus often reducing the pain.

 Like other aspects of coping with arthritis, the keys to a good night's sleep are physical conditioning and experimenting with the suggestions here. Try different positions with your body and pillows to see what works. Some people, for example, find sleeping on their side most comfortable with a pillow between their legs or with a couple of pillows supporting their affected leg. (See Figure 3-6.)

However, you should not sleep *every* night with your knee bent because this position can further tighten and shrink the muscles (known as flexion contracture) of your hip and knee, thereby making the condition worsen over time. Try to sleep with your knee as straight as possible, using pain-relieving medication if necessary. (See the medication section next in this chapter.) However, if your arthritis is quite advanced, stretching doesn't help, and there is no alternative—either you put a pillow under your leg or you don't sleep—then use the pillow.

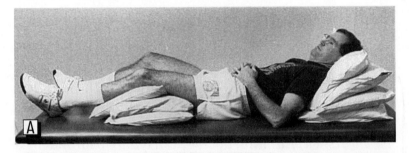

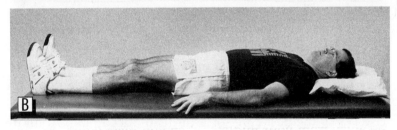

FIGURE 3-6
Lying in Bed and Positioning with Pillows

A. *The most comfortable bed position, but be aware that keeping knees bent over a pillow contributes to the shrinking of hip and thigh muscles.*

B. *The best bed position for a person with hip or knee arthritis.*

A Patient's Perspective: Ron

W HEN MY HIP DETERIORATED to the point that I had to use a pillow, I had best results with the pillow under my knee and lower leg, so that the lower leg was raised and parallel to the bed. Others have told me that they had greater success with the knee bent even more. You need to experiment to see what works best for you.

Use Medication Properly to Control Pain at Night

Although stretching exercises and proper leg and body position can be very effective in decreasing or eliminating pain at night, it may become necessary to take medication to get a good night's sleep. Pain medications, such as those mentioned next in this chapter, taken at bedtime can help control pain and stiffness and facilitate restful sleep. Gentle sleeping pills, prescribed by your physician, can also be helpful.

Arthritis Drug Therapy

Drugs currently available do not change the progression of arthritis.

T HE PRINCIPAL GOAL of drug treatment for arthritis is to relieve your pain so you can maintain as normal a lifestyle as possible. Drugs currently available *do not change the progression of arthritis*, but they can reduce pain and make an unbearable situation manageable.

Successful drug treatment begins with an accurate diagnosis of the cause of pain. This is particularly significant because pain relieving drugs can provide only temporary relief; they are not a cure for the pain. Although muscle pain and stiffness may be reduced by medication, we believe that exercise is still the best cure for arthritis-induced pain. Accurate diagnosis is important for another reason. All drugs have side effects, some of which can be life threatening. Before you take any drug, you want to be certain that it is appropriate for your condition, and that you understand and have considered all the risks and benefits associated with its use.

Remember also that treatment of arthritis with medication is only one aspect of therapy. Exercise, education, and

topical applications (such as ice or heat) are essential therapies that you should use in addition to any drug regimen you
may undertake. Using medication to relieve pain will help
you become more active, which helps you in innumerable
ways. Don't worry about drugs masking your pain, causing
you to potentially harm yourself with activity, for the consequences of being sedentary are far worse.

In general, try exercise, heat or cold, rest, and activity
modification first before adding medication to your therapy
regimen. If pain and stiffness are still bothersome, acetaminophen (which is the active ingredient in Tylenol) is the
safest alternative. If acetaminophen is not effective, discuss
your options with your doctor.

SUPERFICIAL HEAT AND COLD PACKS can help reduce the discomfort of arthritis. Although applications of heat or cold are
not medications, they are medicinal by acting upon the joint
either to increase flexibility and blood flow or to reduce swelling. Although we usually recommend using cold for warm,
swollen joints and heat for chronically stiff joints, there are
no absolute rules.

Applying Heat and Cold

When ice or heat is used, each is more effective if applied for fifteen to twenty minutes and then removed to allow the skin temperature to return to normal. A bag of frozen
peas makes an excellent ice bag that conforms to the knee
joint and warms up as it thaws. Many people find that applying heat prior to exercise and cold immediately afterward is
an effective strategy to limit joint pain. Deep heating treatments, such as ultrasound applied by a therapist or hot wax,
may temporarily reduce pain. However, like all hot and cold
topical applications, the effects do not last long beyond the
initial application.

SOME TOPICAL MEDICATIONS may help relieve arthritis pain.
Capsaicin cream, now available over the counter, is a deriva-
tive of the red pepper plant. It releases and depletes substance
P, which produces pain. Capsaicin cream is applied in a thin

Topical Medications

layer over the painful joint not more than three or four times daily. Capsaicin can burn the first few days it is used. In our experience, it can be helpful for arthritis of the hands and knees, but it is not so effective for hip disease.

Similarly, aspirin creams, such as Aspercreme, can be used to manage pain, but they really only work to the extent that the body absorbs the aspirin. A more effective way to take aspirin is orally. Other topical creams, usually marketed as sports muscle creams, produce a hot feeling when applied to the skin that many people find comforting.

Anti-Inflammatory Drugs

Non-Steroidal Anti-Inflammatories

IN GENERAL, DRUGS ARE PRESCRIBED for two purposes: to re-duce inflammation (anti-inflammatory) and to provide im-mediate pain relief (analgesia).

Drugs that combine pain relief with anti-inflammatory effects are called non-steroidal anti-inflammatories (NSAIDs) and include drugs like ibuprofen, indomethacin, and naproxen. These drugs are often very effective and are available both by prescription (Motrin, Naprosyn, Lodine, Voltaren, Clinoril among others), and over the counter (Ibuprofen, Advil, Nuprin, Mediprin, Motrin-IB). None of these drugs are better than the others, but they all have slightly unique properties. You may find one more tolerable or effective than another. You may need to try several different ones before you discover which is best for you.

Short-acting NSAIDs, such as ibuprofen and naproxen, begin to take effect within an hour of taking the pill. The effect lasts only four to eight hours. Longer acting anti-inflammatories are available by prescription and are to be taken once or twice a day. The twice-a-day medications typically take one to two hours to start working, and are effective up to twelve hours. The once-a-day medications may take from two to four hours to start working, but then last all day.

If you take an anti-inflammatory only once in a while for pain, and you take it when the pain has started, you should take a short-acting one, such as ibuprofen. If, however, you take an anti-inflammatory every day to control your discomfort, then the once-a-day versions may be more useful. Your doctor will advise you about the correct dosage. Bear in mind that usually you will need to take a drug for two weeks before you and your physician can determine its effectiveness.

Aspirin and its derivatives are anti-inflammatory medications that are in a different category from the NSAIDs but also provide pain relief and reduce inflammation. This category of drugs includes aspirin as well as the slightly different compounds, Trilisate and Disalcid. Aspirin has significant analgesic and anti-inflammatory effects, relieving pain and stiffness. Buffered or coated aspirin is usually used to reduce the stomach irritation that aspirin may cause. The benefit of the aspirin derivatives (such as Disalcid) is less frequent stomach irritation compared to aspirin or the NSAIDs. However, many people find them inadequate in relieving pain.

Aspirin and Its Derivatives

Side effects from the anti-inflammatory medications are common. Many people experience adverse gastrointestinal effects such as stomach pains, heartburn, or nausea, which usually means they cannot tolerate the medication. Other potential, but less common, side effects include rashes, ulcers, kidney and liver problems, alterations in mood (like depression), drowsiness, or problems with blood cells. Aspirin and the NSAIDs are well-known causes of stomach ulcers. Some individuals develop ringing in their ears from using large amounts of aspirin or its derivatives.

Side Effects of Anti-Inflammatories

Although significant when they happen, these complications occur in only a small percentage of people who use the drugs. Those with an increased risk of side effects include individuals who take multiple medications, have other serious illnesses, are forgetful, have kidney or liver disease, have a history of stomach or blood disorders, or are elderly. We do not recommend the use of anti-inflammatories if you have a history of stomach ulcers or liver or kidney problems; we prescribe analgesics instead.

Analgesics

Acetaminophen

We recommend acetaminophen as the first drug to use in the treatment of arthritis pain.

ANALGESICS, WHOSE PRIMARY FUNCTION is to reduce pain, include acetaminophen, narcotic derivatives, and some new medications.

Acetaminophen, which is the active ingredient in Tylenol, is a very effective medication for pain, but it does not reduce inflammation. This drug is well tolerated and acts fast to reduce pain. It has been shown to be as effective as the non-steroidal anti-inflammatory drugs (NSAIDs) when used to treat arthritis pain. Acetaminophen has nearly no side effects, but when taken in large doses for a long period of time, it can damage the liver. This usually does not happen if the total daily dosage is less than 3 grams a day. Liver damage can happen with lower doses, however, if combined with alcohol or other medicines that also damage the liver. We strongly recommend acetaminophen as the first drug to use in the treatment of arthritis pain.

Narcotic Derivatives and New Medications

Analgesics, such as acetaminophen, are often combined with codeine and hydrocodone. These stronger medications, which are narcotic derivatives, are available only by prescription. They may be appropriate at times for treating more severe arthritis pain. Side effects may include constipation, dizziness or confusion, and nausea. These drugs also can be addicting.

Tramadol, marketed under the trade name Ultram, is a new pain-relieving agent which is not a narcotic. It can relieve pain while avoiding the addictive potential of the narcotic analgesics. Some reported side effects are drowsiness and confusion.

Steroid Injections

WHEN YOUR ARTHRITIC KNEE is swollen and the pain is severe, a steroid injection may be very helpful. Because the hip is more difficult to inject than the knee, steroid injections are used more frequently for knee pain than for hip pain. Steroid injections may reduce pain quickly and can last from three to six weeks or longer. However, some physicians believe that steroid injections, particularly if used frequently, can accelerate joint deterioration. Moreover, any injection into a joint creates a risk of introducing infection. Therefore, physicians do not recommend more than three steroid injections per year.

Hyaluronic Acid Injections

A NEWLY DEVELOPED SUBSTANCE, hyaluronic acid (currently marketed under the brand names Synvisc or Hyalgan,) has been developed for injection into arthritic knees. Although it has been only recently approved by the Federal Drug Administration for use in the United States, it has been widely used in Europe and Canada. The jelly-like substance, when injected into the knee, acts as a natural buffer for shock absorption and facilitates smooth joint motion. The substance covers and deadens nerve endings, thus reducing pain. Hyaluronic acid is derived from naturally occurring chemicals in cartilage and dissolves naturally in a short period of time. There do not appear to be any short-term side effects from the preparation. Its use appears promising for the treatment of a wide variety of joint problems.

The Cost of Drugs

ALL THE PRESCRIPTION anti-inflammatory drugs are *expensive*. It costs about two dollars a day for treatment at the prescribed doses. Ask your doctor or nurse about ways of getting discounted prescriptions if you have limited financial resources. Non-prescription drugs such as acetaminophen, aspirin, and the generic forms of ibuprofen and naproxen are much less expensive and, for many, are just as effective as the brand-name arthritis medications.

A Patient's Perspective: Ron

FROM MY PERSPECTIVE, drugs were a double-edged sword. They were beneficial in that they relieved my pain, especially during the middle part of my struggle with arthritis, which is the point at which I was constantly aware that I had the disease, but surgery was not yet necessary. The downside to using drugs, in addition to the side effects, was that the necessity of taking the drugs became yet another annoying signal of the inevitable decline of my joint. Caught in the iron grip of the disease, I came both to depend on the drugs and to resent them at the same time.

This two-sided aspect of drug therapy can be a blessing, however. I say that because drugs almost always are a means of postponing the inevitable, and that is very important to bear in mind. As your arthritis progresses, the pain will always return and will have to be dealt with in some other way. If you do not keep this point well in mind, you may find yourself increasing the dosage of the drug you are taking without your doctor's advice, or you may begin shopping for different drugs because you believe the drug you are taking now no longer works, but that perhaps another will. Don't let yourself be caught in these mindsets. Drugs will help you make the transition from the early stages of arthritis to its later stages when surgery may be required, but they are not a cure. Your disease will progress. Increasing the dosage of the drug you are taking may provide a little more relief, but it also increases dramatically the risks of side effects. You should talk to your doctor about the proper dosage and stay within his or her guidelines.

Shopping for a new drug is also likely to prove ineffectual, and has its risks as well. As your pain returns, it almost surely will be from the continuing degeneration of your joint or muscles, which no drug can stop. My problem was not that the drugs I was taking were no longer working, but that my hip was deteriorating to the point where something else was required—surgery. If you need a drug to treat your arthritis pain, don't overlook the fact that you also need exercise. Using drugs is probably *less* effective in the long run than exercising appropriately in making life bearable. Also remember that every time you take a new drug, you risk new side effects. The more you take, the higher the risk. So if you have had some success with a drug, stick with it at the levels prescribed. When your situation begins to deteriorate, it will be time to consider other options.

With both my hips, I had success with only one drug, naproxen. This is not a commercial for naproxen, however. It just so happened that every other drug I tried had one of two side effects, which David and Vicky's discussion understate, in my view. The first was serious gastrointestinal problems, constipation, and the resultant hemorrhoidal problems. The second was that, with the two drugs that I tried before I settled on naproxen, I went into a state of clinical depression. I found myself listless, with no energy and no interest in anything. I had an almost physical sense of being tied or weighed down, as though every movement was a struggle. When I realized this, I quit taking the drug, and within a few days I was emotionally back to normal.

The side effects that the doctors talk about are real, and of course I can only relate the ones that had physical or emotional manifestations for me. These side effects are idiosyncratic to individual patients, however. Some drugs affect some people in some ways, and other drugs affect other people in other ways. Naproxen worked for me, but it may not for you. Fortunately, there are enough alternatives so that with careful experimentation in consultation with your doctors, you should be able to find a drug that provides relief with no discernible side effects.

One final point about drugs. Some side effects of drugs cannot be detected through your own self-observation, such as damage to internal organs. Blood tests are available that indicate if a drug you are taking is causing undesirable metabolic changes. Consequently, you should consult an internist or general practitioner whenever you undergo a drug regimen that may last for longer than a few months.

A VARIETY OF ALTERNATIVE TREATMENTS and medicines are used for arthritis that you should also be aware of. Some of these strategies are useful, others can be potentially harmful and expensive, while still others are simply unproved. We feel it's important to understand the risks and benefits of any treatment available. (See Table 3-5.)

MEDITATION HAS BEEN USED for centuries to reduce stress and manage pain and is an acceptable complement to exercise and medication for treating arthritis pain. Similarly, massage can reduce pain and tension and may help improve sleep. Another relaxation and pain-relieving technique is biofeedback, which involves the use of sensory equipment to monitor your heart, blood pressure, and muscle responses to help

Alternative Treatments and Medicines

Meditation, Massage, and Biofeedback

you control involuntary responses to stress, muscle spasms, and pain. Biofeedback is usually taught by pain psychologists, nurses, or physical therapists. It is now a quite well-accepted and effective pain management technique.

Acupuncture

ACUPUNCTURE TREATMENT inserts thin needles into the skin on specific points of the body. The goal is to restore *qi*, or vital energy, which when out of balance (according to Far-Eastern practitioners), leads to illness and pain. Acupuncture has been widely studied and is known to be safe and sometimes effective. Some evidence exists that shows acupuncture to be useful in relieving pain from arthritis. There are increasing numbers of practitioners of acupuncture in the United States. This treatment has become more readily available and acknowledged by traditional medical care providers.

Chiropractic Manipulation

CHIROPRACTIC TREATMENT MAY ALSO BE complementary to traditional methods of arthritis treatment. Chiropractors believe that, through regular joint manipulation, pain and even arthritis itself can be eliminated; however, medical doctors strongly disagree. You should know that *chiropractic treatment may be harmful for individuals with unstable joints, severe*

TABLE 3-5: Commonly Asked-About Alternative Treatments for Arthritis

Helpful	Unproven but Promising	Unproven	Harmful
Massage	Glucosamine	Dimethyl Sulfoxide (DMSO)	Bee stings
Meditation	Chondroitin Sulphate	Golden Creme (histamine dihydrochloride)	Black pearl
Biofeedback	Vitamin D		Chinese black balls
Acupuncture	Special diet (such as fish with high Omega-3 fatty acids)	Copper and zinc	
Chiropractic		Vitamins B and C	
Capsaicin		Shark cartilage	

osteoporosis, spinal stenosis, or instability. Chiropractors are not schooled in medical diagnosis; thus, if you are experiencing severe pain, you should see a medical doctor before trying a chiropractor.

HEALTH FOOD STORES and some drugstores abound with unproven medicines, herbs, and vitamins for arthritis treatment. For example, black pearl or Chinese black balls (*chuifong tuokuwan*) are distributed as an herbal remedy which provides dramatic relief for arthritis. This compound is illegal in the United States and contains some very strong medications, including steroids and tranquilizers. It has even killed some people.

Unproven Medications

Some practitioners of alternative medicine suggest that bee venom, administered through daily bee stings, will relieve the pain of arthritis. There is no proof that this works. In addition, some people are highly allergic to bee stings or can develop an allergy, which makes this treatment potentially very dangerous.

Dimethyl Sulfoxide (DMSO), legally obtained in some states, is a very controversial treatment for arthritis. Studies of its effectiveness are incomplete and have yielded mixed results. Some studies have suggested DMSO reduces pain and inflammation of certain types of arthritis, while others have shown that it may speed up joint deterioration. DMSO has many side effects, including various allergic reactions, diarrhea, nausea, and drowsiness.

Shark's cartilage has received a substantial amount of media attention for its purported influence in preventing arthritis. But no conclusive studies to date have proved it to be safe or effective.

Several lubricants are available to treat arthritis, all of which are unproven. For example, Golden Creme, which contains histamine dihydrochloride, is a topical cream touted to dramatically reduce pain and swelling.

In conclusion we must emphasize that *there are no studies proving the effectiveness of any of these treatments, or documenting*

their potentially negative side effects. When asked about the use of these unproven medications, *as long as there are no known or conceivable ill effects*, we do not discourage patients from trying them as long as they continue to use the proven strategies we have described.

Diet and Nutrition

ALTHOUGH NO EVIDENCE SUGGESTS that any dietary strategy will reduce the symptoms of arthritis, your diet is important. A well-balanced, healthy diet maintains an optimal immune system, energy level, and capacity to exercise. Copper, zinc, and vitamins B, C, and D have all been proposed as anti-arthritis supplements, but no nutritional supplements have shown specific benefits.

Glucosamine and chondroitin sulphate are two nutritional supplements which have been promoted as cures for arthritis, but they are not regulated by the U.S. Food and Drug Administration. Both are said to assist in repairing and maintaining cartilage. Recently, these supplements have been promoted as a cure for arthritis. Although some European studies have indicated that these substances may be useful, their testing is not yet complete. At this point, they should not be considered a cure for arthritis, and their use should not replace the current recommended strategies of weight control, exercise, proper nutrition, and the use of anti-inflammatory medications.

Overcome the Emotional Issues of Arthritis

MANY EMOTIONAL ISSUES ARISE when a patient develops arthritis. Two of the most debilitating are those related to problems with sexual relationships and to depression.

SEXUAL PROBLEMS ARE A COMMON RESULT of arthritis. In fact, most people with arthritis of the hips and knees experience some difficulties in their sexual relationships. First, joint pain and stiffness limit mobility and interfere with a wide variety of sexual expression. The pain from a hip with arthritis is made worse with hip rotation, such as that which occurs during sexual intercourse in the missionary position. Joint pain and stiffness are often worst at the end of a long day—just when intimacy with your partner is desired. It is often difficult enough to find a comfortable position to sleep in, let alone one to make love in. Unless you learn to deal with these issues, you may find that your marital relationship becomes seriously strained.

Second, many people with arthritis report a reduction in their sexual drive and responsiveness. This results from many factors. Fatigue, whether from painful, sleepless nights or the extra work of just living with arthritis, naturally reduces libido. Medications are also known to directly reduce sexual drive and function. Although using medications to reduce pain may improve your physical ability to perform sexually, their use can often hinder the urge to do so.

Thus you may feel inadequate and worry about not meeting your partner's needs. You may also feel guilty about not behaving like a "normal" partner. You may even become fearful of losing your lover.

Your partner is also likely to have concerns and fears about your sexual relationship. He or she may be reluctant to make love because of the fear of causing you pain. Your partner may feel inhibited by the need to discuss specific sexual positions and may feel that the spontaneity of your sexual relationship is or will be lost. He or she may feel frustrated and annoyed with the change in the sexual relationship that your arthritis has produced. Your partner may even believe that your lack of interest in sexual intercourse actually reflects a lack of interest in him or her.

You can use several methods to lessen difficulties with sexual expression. Understand and accept that these problems are *normal*. Exploring the issues and looking for solutions with your partner will not only improve your communication, but may actually be enjoyable. Trying new positions or different methods of achieving sexual satisfaction is not abnormal or depraved. The whole idea is to find a mutually satisfying

Sexual Relationships

Understand Your Partner's Concerns

Discover Solutions

*Address These
Issues with
Your Doctor*

method of sexual expression which keeps both of you fulfilled and happy. (See Table 3-6.)

If finding these solutions is difficult for you and your partner to do on your own, discuss the subject with your doctor. Sometimes simple changes in the treatment of your arthritis may remedy the problem. For instance, changing a particular medication may improve mobility of your hips and knees.

Discussing these issues with your doctor may not be easy for you. Although researchers have suggested that up to three-quarters of patients with arthritis want their doctors to be concerned and ask about their sexual issues, only a limited number report that their doctors actually ask about such problems. Why don't doctors ask about sexual problems resulting from arthritis? Perhaps it is because medical schools offer limited training in human sexuality. Perhaps physicians assume this issue is none of their business. Or maybe they believe their patients will bring up the issue if it is important. Most likely, they—like you—are embarrassed to broach the topic. Like many other aspects of your arthritis care, you may have to take the initiative to get what you need, deserve, and want.

Often, just being educated about what is or isn't safe to do can resolve any guilt or fear which may be inhibiting you or your partner from enjoying sex. It may be that you and your partner would benefit from sexual counseling—by a nurse, psychologist, social worker, or family therapist. If,

 TABLE 3-6: Planning for Better Sex with Arthritis

❏ Plan for sex at a time of day when you generally feel best.
❏ If you take a pain relief medication, time it so its effect will occur during love-making.
❏ Pace your activities during the day so you avoid extreme fatigue.
❏ Relax your joints with stretching exercises (see Chapter 8).
❏ Take a warm bath or shower before sex to relax and soothe you.

after you discuss the topic with your doctor, you need or would like more information, ask your doctor to refer you to a skilled counselor. Just remember that sexual problems as a consequence of arthritis are real, common, and important. If you acknowledge the issues early on, you can often find simple, effective solutions which will allow you to continue to enjoy a satisfying sexual life.

A Patient's Perspective: Ron

SEXUAL DYSFUNCTION RESULTS FROM INCREASING DISCOMFORT as arthritis progresses. In many, many cases, the response is to avoid what hurts, even if that means foregoing pleasurable and meaningful activity. I strongly urge you not to let this happen to you. You can maintain a happy and satisfying sexual relationship throughout the entire course of arthritis. It does require some effort, but thankfully it can be highly rewarding. The secret to maintaining satisfying sexual relationships is simply communication with your partner. Share your problem and search for a solution together. If you talk with your partner about the need to modify your sexual practices because of your discomfort, you can begin a fun and gratifying search for a mutually satisfactory solution. And I can almost guarantee that you will find one if you look.

Another reason to be open with your partner about the effect of arthritis on your sexual relationship is that he or she may not know that your apparent declining interest in sex is caused by pain rather than emotional distance. You, in other words, may not be the only one suffering because of your disease, and often you can alleviate the emotional pain of your partner by being frank about your physical discomfort. Nothing could be more important. You have enough problems with the physical side of arthritis. You do not need to compound them by needlessly generating emotional difficulties. Let your physical problems bring you closer to those you love rather than drive you apart.

Depression

DEPRESSION IS A MAJOR HEALTH PROBLEM in the United States and is common in people with chronic conditions such as arthritis. Studies of persons with osteoarthritis of the hip or knee indicate that up to twenty percent may have symptoms of depression. In older persons, especially, depression is underdiagnosed and undertreated.

Depression is disabling because it reduces your ability to perform even the simplest tasks, impairs social functioning, and can make your arthritis pain feel worse. Depression may be more than just a feeling of being blue. It can manifest itself in many ways, such as changes in thinking, an inability to concentrate, changes in behavior such as irritability or agitation, or physical changes such as sleep disturbances, fatigue, weight loss or gain, reduced libido, indigestion, or increased general body pain. In addition, loss of self-esteem, loss of interest in daily activities, or unusual feelings of anxiety may also be signs of depression.

Fortunately, treatment for depression by counseling and sometimes antidepressant medication has proven to be effective. Many persons' symptoms improve in just a short while. Patients with arthritis may be particularly prone to becoming depressed. The treatment of your arthritis may depend on the successful treatment of this depression.

A Patient's Perspective: Ron

YOU MAY FIND YOURSELF STRUGGLING with arthritis, and you may not be able to do some things as quickly and easily as other people. You may at some point have a limp that will bring attention to yourself. You might worry or be embarrassed about these things. Again, these are natural and unavoidable feelings. Don't let them discourage you from engaging with the world; you should be living life to the fullest. To help you do so, let me relate my own experience, for I eventually came to realize that most people sympathized with my difficulties.

If I had trouble getting onto a bus, or if it took me a bit longer to get in or out of a car, those waiting for me never complained. When I first started limping and was questioned about it, I often did not give straight answers because I did not want to be the object of pity. But I found that, when I began being more honest and open about my condition, invariably my answer was met with good-natured sympathy. Those of us suffering from arthritis can easily become self-absorbed and overlook the fact that everyone else has problems of their own. I discovered that I was not the only person with an imperfect body, and behind that discovery lies a tremendous reservoir of humanity. Our bodies are constantly growing and decaying. In some of us, that fact is just more obvious than in others.

So it's okay to feel a little sorry for yourself, but then take control of your life. Throw off the sack cloth and put on your exercise clothes. You can handle this problem, just like you've been able to handle most of life's problems. You just happen to have to deal with something that many others don't, but don't forget that every life is unique. Arthritis is no picnic, but neither is it metastatic cancer or Alzheimer's disease. Its symptoms can be controlled for a long time, and very successful surgery is available if and when necessary. Don't allow it to control you. Your arthritis is merely another aspect of your uniqueness as a person. Don't let it drive you away from people; use it to better understand yourself and others. You are the master, not some joint that is giving out too soon. And don't forget it.

Conclusion

As we have shown, every activity that you do, or that you did and would like to do again, can be modified to accommodate your changing physical condition. You don't have to continue struggling to do everything as you did before. Don't think that somehow changing your behavior is an undesirable concession to your affliction; exactly the opposite is true. What makes us human is the ability to change our environment to suit our needs. As your needs continue to change, modify your environment accordingly to facilitate your activity. All you need to do is think about what is difficult and what you can do to make it easier. If you can't come up with a solution yourself, ask the advice of an occupational therapist or your doctor.

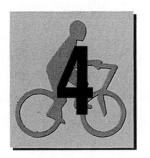

BUILDING to the DECISION to OPERATE

THERE MAY COME A TIME when the pain or the loss of function in your hip or knee has become so great that your only option to eliminate the pain and restore function is surgery, whether relatively minor or major. Surgical options include arthroscopy, osteotomy, and arthrodesis, as well as total joint replacement. The appropriateness of each method depends on the cause and extent of your arthritis, and we describe each form of surgery in this chapter.

Most persons with osteoarthritis will not need joint replacement surgery. We devote the most attention to it here, however, because deciding whether and when to undergo hip or knee replacement is by far the most difficult and the most important decision that you may need to make.

The decision is difficult because the criteria used to determine when a joint replacement is necessary are not absolute and vary from person to person. Individuals vary in how they perceive pain, how the loss of function will affect them, and how willing they are to take risks.

The decision is important because joint replacement procedures include all the risks that accompany major surgical undertakings. Like many surgical procedures, total joint replacements are not always completely successful. Recovery from total joint replacements can take as short as four weeks or as long as six months. Although unsuccessful joint replacements can be effectively exchanged, the revision surgery (that is, the replacement of the earlier prosthetic joint) is complex and presents more possibilities for failure than the initial joint replacement. Therefore, you need to weigh carefully the risks and benefits of total joint surgery before deciding to undergo the procedure.

Your Responsibility as Patient

YOU SHOULD BECOME AS INFORMED as possible about your condition, especially if your hip or knee is beginning to degenerate to the point where exercise and medication are unable to control it. Your local library will be able to provide you with basic information, and your physician should be able to name some articles on the issues relevant to your condition. Reference librarians at your local library and at a medical library near you will be happy to help you obtain these and related materials. And the internet is a good source for information, but consult your physician about the accuracy and reliability of what you find there.

Obviously you can't become an orthopedic specialist, but you can learn a remarkable amount in a short time. In particular, you can learn enough to ask more intelligent questions of your doctors, and thus get better, more complete answers. Given the importance of the decisions you may have to make, this would be time well spent.

ALTHOUGH JOINT REPLACEMENT SURGERY is usually appropriate when patients have clinical symptoms and x-ray evidence of advanced arthritis, you and your orthopedic physician should not consider such surgery until you have tried all the non-surgical methods to control pain and loss of function (see Chapter 3) and found them no longer to be successful. A joint with advanced arthritis is not necessarily so painful or disabling that joint replacement surgery is necessary. A saying among physicians who care for patients with arthritis is that "you don't walk on your x-rays." *Many patients with advanced arthritis of the hip or knee function at very high levels with relatively tolerable pain.*

The primary responsibility of physicians who care for arthritic patients, including those with advanced arthritis, is to prescribe and supervise an effective non-operative treatment program. As we explained in Chapter 3, essential to a program's success is a patient's understanding that continuing to be active on an arthritic joint is not detrimental to that joint. Many patients and, unfortunately, many physicians have the misconception that activity, including relatively vigorous exercise, somehow hastens the deterioration of an arthritic joint. In fact, the opposite is true. Joints that are not kept active are usually more painful and stiffer than joints that are kept active and strong.

Three aspects of a non-surgical treatment program for patients considering total joint surgery are exercise, medication, and weight control.

EXERCISE IS THE CORNERSTONE of all non-surgical treatment programs for arthritis. Exercise improves the capacity and efficiency of a joint and can often reduce or eliminate pain within it. The rationale for using exercise as a strategy to control arthritis is described in Chapter 3 and detailed in Chapter 8. It is important for you to realize that just because you have a moderately or severely diseased hip or knee does not mean you should stop exercising. We see many patients whose x-rays show their arthritis to be advanced, some of whom

Non-Surgical Ways to Control Pain and Loss of Function

Exercise

have been told that they need joint replacement, but who can adequately control their arthritis symptoms when they follow an appropriate exercise program. Also, should you eventually need to undergo joint replacement surgery, you will recover much more quickly if you have been exercising diligently.

Medications

MEDICATIONS ARE ANOTHER ESSENTIAL COMPONENT of a non-surgical treatment program. Although we have detailed in Chapter 3 the types of medications used to treat arthritis, we must emphasize here the role they play for joint replacement candidates.

Often persons who become candidates for this type of surgery tend to take their medications less systematically than usual. Perhaps they are obtaining less than satisfactory relief from the medications and realize that the upcoming surgery will probably eliminate the need for them. If you find this is happening to you, remember that it is very important to maintain your medication so you can be as pain-free as possible before surgery. By obtaining pain relief, you are more likely to sleep satisfactorily, to continue your exercise program, and to maintain your appetite. If the anti-inflammatory agents or acetaminophen-containing drugs are not adequately controlling your pain, you may require a narcotic-containing analgesic.

Weight Control

WEIGHT CONTROL IS ANOTHER FACTOR critical to controlling the symptoms of arthritis. You may be particularly uncomfortable in the weeks before surgery and find exercise difficult. You may also be more anxious than usual as you anticipate the surgery. Reduced levels of activity and increased anxiety often lead to weight gain. It is important not to gain or lose weight just before undergoing surgery because being in a balanced nutritional state enables your tissues to heal faster immediately after your surgery.

Many patients wonder if weighing more than their ideal weight will adversely affect their surgery. Sometimes patients feel guilty that their weight may have caused or aggravated their arthritis. There is no evidence that this is true.

Operating on an overweight patient is more difficult techni-
cally but will probably not adversely affect the outcome of a
procedure. Some surgeons insist that patients weigh less than
a certain amount—two hundred pounds is a commonly
quoted figure—before they will carry out the procedure. Our
approach is to encourage patients to lose weight before the
procedure if they need and want to. However, we do not believe that total joint surgery should be denied to those who
need it if their weight is the only prohibiting factor. If you are
concerned about how your being overweight may affect the
surgery, discuss this with your surgeon well beforehand.

When exercise, medications, and weight control are no
longer able to control the pain and disability of arthritis, we
counsel our patients to consider surgery and sometimes joint
replacement.

Many patients who have been advised to consider surgery are well over seventy years of age. Yet because
of their advanced age, many wrongly believe that they should
not consider joint replacement. They may have been told by
their doctor that they are too old and should consider surgery only as a last resort. Sometimes they know people who
have not done well with surgery and conclude that they might
not either.

The fact is that healthy older persons, including those over
eighty years of age, do just as well as younger persons undergoing hip or knee replacement surgery. The risk of death, of
complications, or of having an unsuccessful outcome is not any
more than that for younger patients. In addition, older patients
should rarely require revision surgery and thus do not need to
anticipate it. Older patients have much more to fear from the
likely complications of the progressive inactivity that accom-
panies severe arthritis. Inactivity in older persons, more so than
in younger patients, accelerates deterioration of heart and lung
function as well as musculoskeletal function.

Concerns of Older Patients

The pain from severe arthritis of the hip and knee can cause loss of sleep and appetite. Fatigue and malnutrition are poorly tolerated by and potentially dangerous for older people. A decline in activity may lead to depression, which in turn may lead to a decline in overall health. This downward spiral is why we encourage our patients to seriously consider joint replacement surgery once non-surgical approaches become inadequate or unsuccessful.

The decision about surgery is a difficult one. Educate yourself as well as you can about the potential risks and benefits of surgery so you can take those factors into account as you contemplate how bearable your physical condition is.

Less Invasive Surgical Methods

IF YOU ARE NO LONGER responding to non-surgical treatment of your arthritis, but you don't need a total joint replacement, you might be a candidate for an alternative, more limited surgery. Depending on the extent of your arthritis, these surgical methods can, in some cases, prevent the development of severe arthritis. In other cases, especially if you are a younger patient with severe arthritis, they can enable you to delay total joint replacement surgery as long as possible with the hope that new technological developments may provide devices that will last the rest of your lifetime. Several such surgical procedures are available.

Arthroscopy (Primarily for Knees)

THE SURGICAL PROCEDURE OF GREATEST appeal as an alternative to total joint replacement surgery is arthroscopy. It is minimally invasive and can be performed as an outpatient procedure, which means that patients can return to their routine functions a few days after surgery. Arthroscopy has a definite role in the treatment of osteoarthritis of the knee, but it is limited in treating osteoarthritis of the hip.

As osteoarthritis progresses, a number of changes occur within the knee joint that are amenable to arthroscopic surgical treatment. The meniscus or the anterior cruciate ligament may start to fray and may even tear, causing pain, locking, or giving way. Or pieces of articular cartilage or osteophytes (spurs) may break off and become loose within the knee joint, causing symptoms very similar to those of a torn or frayed meniscus. These symptoms can be very effectively treated by arthroscopic surgery.

Arthroscopic surgery is most frequently performed on patients with a history of generally mild knee symptoms who experience a significant increase in pain, swelling, and loss of knee mobility and function. Most patients who develop these new symptoms can be successfully treated non-surgically with a brief period of reduced activity, medication, and modified exercises, such as non–weight-bearing, strengthening exercises. If the new symptoms do not respond to this treatment program within a few weeks, arthroscopic surgery may be indicated as an option.

In arthroscopic surgery, the surgeon inserts into the affected joint a narrow tube that contains a fiber-optic system of lenses (the arthroscope) for a video camera that he or she uses to see inside the joint. Tools, some power driven, are inserted into the joint through incisions the size of that used for the arthroscope, where they smooth rough surfaces, remove loose pieces of tissue, or cut away uneven edges of structures like menisci or ligaments. The surgeon uses fluid to irrigate and distend the joint during the procedure. (See Figure 4-1.)

Although arthroscopic surgery can be performed under local anesthesia, the procedure is more commonly carried out under a regional (epidural or spinal) or general anesthetic. Patients typically leave the hospital a few hours after the procedure, and they usually need to use crutches or a cane for a few days afterward.

Arthroscopic surgery can be very helpful for eliminating the source of pain and dysfunction in an arthritic joint. However, the effectiveness of this surgery is greatest in joints that have relatively mild arthritis. The more advanced the degeneration, the less effective the procedure is likely to be and the shorter the duration of symptom relief. Arthroscopic

FIGURE 4-1
Arthroscopy

A. *The medial (inside) femoral-tibial compartment of the right knee, viewed through an arthroscope. Both the femur and the tibia have severe arthritis. The meniscus has a degenerative tear related to the arthritis.*

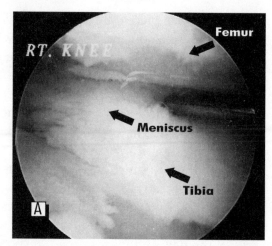

surgery does not alter the progression of osteoarthritis. Thus, arthroscopic surgery is not a substitute for total joint surgery.

Many patients with relatively advanced arthritis hope that the minimally invasive arthroscopic surgery procedure might provide some symptom relief and postpone the need for total joint replacement surgery. In our experience, these patients who proceed with the surgery are usually very disappointed and discouraged by the results. We recommend that patients who have more advanced arthritis forgo such surgery and continue their non-surgical treatment program until they are ready for total joint replacement surgery.

Osteotomy (For Knees or Hips)

OSTEOTOMY IS A SURGICAL PROCEDURE that corrects the malalignment of a joint. A mal-aligned joint is likely to degenerate more quickly and to be more painful than a correctly aligned joint. The goals of an osteotomy, therefore, are to realign and straighten the bones around the joint so the stresses on the joint will be close to normal, and to reduce the accompanying pain and loss of function. To accomplish these goals, the osteotomy procedure actually breaks and removes a wedge of bone from the arthritic hip or knee.

Deformities of the hip or knee can predispose the joints to arthritis and become more pronounced and obvious as the arthritis progresses. For example, a person who is bowlegged will have increased pressure on the inside of the knee

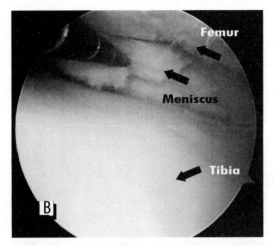

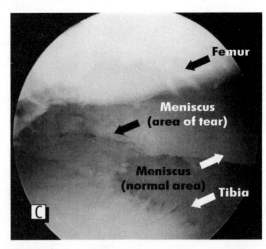

joint when he or she walks. This person may find that simply walking is painful and awkward. Correction of the deformity may reduce the pain and make walking less awkward even if he or she does not have degenerative arthritis. If the person does have some arthritis in the bowed knee, and has pain and loss of function as a result, the correction of the deformity may be even more effective in reducing the pain and loss of function. (See Figure 4-2.) Another common deformity of the knee that can predispose a person to osteoarthritis is knock-knee.

B. The torn meniscal fragment has been partially removed from the right knee.

C. The torn meniscal fragment has been removed from the right knee.

The goal of an osteotomy of the tibia (one of the two bones of the lower leg), then, is to correct the bowlegged or knock-knee deformities and distribute the pressure more evenly throughout the knee joint.

Although most apparent in the knee, pre-existing deformities around the hip joint, such as childhood hip conditions, can also predispose individuals to degenerative arthritis relatively early in adulthood. For instance, in dysplasia of the hip, a relatively common condition in women, the acetabulum (cup) may be incorrectly directed. This acetabular malalignment results in increased pressure on a portion of the cup and head of the femur (the thigh bone). The goal of a pelvic osteotomy is to correct this direction of the acetabulum and redistribute the pressure over the femoral head and cup more uniformly.

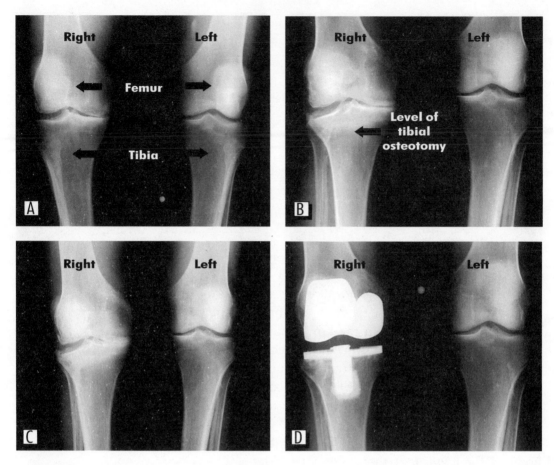

FIGURE 4-2
Osteotomy

In some cases osteotomy, which corrects mal-alignment of a joint, can prevent the need for further surgery. But <u>in most cases, because osteoarthritis continues to cause the joint to degenerate, an osteotomy merely postpones the need for total joint replacement</u>, as shown here.

A. A forty-year-old athletic man with moderate arthritis on his right knee, before a tibial osteotomy.

B. Two years after the tibial osteotomy, the arthritis has progressed, but he still participates in sports.

C. Eight years after the osteotomy, his arthritis is now severe, and he can no longer do routine activities comfortably.

D. Two years after his total knee replacement, he has returned to non–high impact athletic activities.

Osteotomy is usually reserved for very young patients to delay joint replacement surgery. The indications for osteotomy are fairly rare. In the knee, for example, only one side of the joint can be arthritic if the procedure is to succeed.

Osteotomy is performed under either epidural or general anesthesia and requires a short hospital stay. Depending upon the location of the osteotomy, the broken bone may require six to twenty-four weeks to heal. After this recovery period, patients need to exercise aggressively to restore joint mobility and strength. During the period of healing, patients may have to avoid placing all of their weight on the extremity. Afterward, patients walk with crutches bearing only partial weight on their affected leg for four to six weeks. Because the osteotomy for the treatment or prevention of arthritis is performed near a joint, it is important that therapy be started shortly after the procedure to assure that joint motion is not lost. Some types of fixation used to hold the osteotomy fragments in place, such as an external fixator or metal plate, have to be removed at some point after the operation.

Thus, an osteotomy is an operation of reasonably significant complexity and size that requires a number of weeks or months for complete recovery. It is a substantially more involved operation than an arthroscopy. Like an arthroscopy, however, an osteotomy offers patients the prospect that joint replacement can be postponed for some period of time. Patients who have had successful osteotomies can return to heavy labor or running sports if they need or want to.

Osteotomies, then, are most suitable for patients with a significant deformity near a joint in which there is relatively little arthritis. Younger patients usually have better, longer-lasting results than older patients. Osteotomies of the knee usually postpone the need for a total knee replacement for five to ten years, though occasionally patients obtain significant relief for much longer periods. Osteotomies of the hip are most commonly performed in children, adolescents, and young adults who have deformities caused by childhood hip diseases. These patients usually do not need total hip replacements until their forties, fifties, or sixties.

Arthrodesis (For Knees or Hips)

PERSONS WHO ARE VERY YOUNG or who have had a serious or recurring joint infection may not be appropriate candidates for joint replacement but may still require surgery to alleviate the pain from a severely degenerated joint. Arthrodesis, or fusion, of the hip or knee joint is one method of relieving severe joint pain. After the surgery, however, joint motion is entirely eliminated. The patient is left with a painless but rigid joint.

This technique is used quite frequently for treating severe arthritis of the fingers, toes, and ankles. However, the loss of motion that necessarily results from fusing a previously mobile joint makes the usefulness of the arthrodesis procedure relatively limited in the treatment of arthritis of the hip and knee. Patients who have arthritis of these joints are rarely willing to give up motion in return for pain relief.

Factors in Considering Joint Replacement Surgery

HIP OR KNEE REPLACEMENT is indicated when pain and functional limitations begin to significantly reduce your quality of life. Each of us has a different tolerance for pain and disability. Some patients are so fearful of the potential risks of general anesthesia and surgery that they would rather live with pain and limited mobility. Each person must decide if and when surgery is needed.

Although younger, healthier persons may be less tolerant of the limited mobility associated with advanced arthritic joints, older persons actually may be more at risk from the negative impacts of limited mobility. For example, an eighty-five year old may suffer the disastrous consequences of immobility from arthritis and develop such problems as pneumonia and heart disease. These may ultimately result in the person's inability to care for him- or herself. Older persons are also more likely to develop the side effects of the medicines used to control arthritis pain. For these reasons, we frequently encourage our older patients not to wait as long as younger individuals to undergo surgery.

THE DECISION TO OPERATE is complex and includes a careful weighing of risks and benefits. You need to understand many specific aspects of joint replacement when building to the decision to operate. You must understand the expected physical and functional outcome of the surgery and the risks of complications and implant failure. You will want to find an experienced surgeon with whom you are comfortable developing a long-term relationship. Discuss with your surgeon the known and theoretical benefits of different types of implants. You will need to time your surgery so that the short-term disability you experience after the operation occurs when it is least disruptive to you, your family, and your work. Take time to understand the financial implications of surgery, and before surgery make sure you have resolved any questions about reimbursement for your care (inpatient, outpatient, and home care). You should also familiarize yourself with hospital procedures so you can plan around the restrictions.

Risks and Benefits

HIP AND KNEE REPLACEMENTS are dramatically successful procedures. For those with osteoarthritis, long-term outcome studies report that more than ninety-five percent of patients who have had the surgery rate their outcome as good or excellent. In our experience, over eighty percent of patients are completely pain-free after surgery, while an additional sixteen to seventeen percent have only mild, non–function impacting pain. All of these patients note substantial improvement over their pre-operative condition. About three or four percent of patients are unhappy with their outcome, for a variety of reasons.

Death is an almost unheard of complication of joint replacement surgery. The orthopedic literature reports a mortality rate of .5 percent in persons older than age sixty-five undergoing joint replacement. These patients are usually frail, with significant heart, lung, or vascular disease. Complications of joint replacement surgery, discussed in Chapter 5, are relatively rare.

Expected Physical and Functional Outcomes after Surgery

After surgery and physical therapy, most people can walk without an assistive device for long distances. With practice, they can eventually climb stairs in the usual manner. With good rehabilitation, most people are able to return to a high level of physical functioning, such as golfing, hiking, gardening, and other activities.

Post-Operative Disability and Recovery

Hip and knee replacement surgery does require an extensive post-operative period of recovery. After an initial four- or five-day acute care hospital stay, most people are discharged with home health care nursing and physical therapy. They then progress to outpatient therapy. Joint replacement requires dedication to exercise for *at least six months after surgery* to ensure an excellent outcome. Many patients report that they do not feel like themselves for up to a year after surgery. Sleeping patterns may not return to normal for a year. Most people return to driving a car six to eight weeks after surgery and can also return to work around that time.

Those who are frail, have had extensive surgery, or are older and live alone may require more inpatient care than others. These patients typically transfer to a rehabilitation unit within the same hospital or in a neighboring rehabilitation hospital, or they may go to a community-based nursing home. They may be hospitalized one or two weeks or longer and will receive rehabilitative therapy until they reach the level of independence required for them to go home.

Expected Longevity of an Implant

Orthopedic technology is advancing rapidly. Every year, cement techniques, implant design, and surgical techniques improve. Therefore, postponing surgery may enable you to reap substantial benefits from the development of new technology. However, current hip and knee replacements should last fifteen to twenty years or longer. Because we expect these implants to last about twenty years, younger patients with a life expectancy greater than twenty years must consider the risk of future revision surgery in their decision to undergo total joint replacement surgery.

Conversely, the possibility of new developments must be weighed against the very real daily losses experienced when arthritis is progressing. It may make more sense for a thirty-five year old to wait for new technologies than a sixty-five year old. Current technology can give a sixty-five year old a prosthetic joint which will last his or her lifetime. We cannot yet promise that for a thirty-five year old. (Chapter 7 discusses revision surgery further.)

A Patient's Perspective: Ron

How Did I Decide to Replace My Left Hip?

To HELP YOU BETTER UNDERSTAND and evaluate your options, let me describe my experience and explain my own thinking about the question of whether and when to operate.

I HAVE BEEN QUITE FORTUNATE in having received exceptional medical care in my struggle with arthritis, but there was one time when I felt like throttling my surgeon, David Stulberg. As my left hip deteriorated I began investigating hip replacement surgery, through both lengthy discussions with David and my own research efforts in the library. I searched for the answer to one question in particular, which was when I should have my left hip replaced. Every source I consulted, including David, said the same thing: Surgery is sensible when your condition begins to interfere with the quality of life or when it substantially impairs the quality of life. But how would I know when that was? When I talked with David, he would ask, "And does your pain still respond to aspirin (and later naproxen)? Are you able to sleep at night?" Early on my answers were yes. This would generate another smile from David and a comment that it wasn't time yet. That's when I felt the throttling urge come on. I wanted to know how and when I would know.

Still, even though I was frustrated with these interactions, I also knew that David was correct when he said I was not yet ready for surgery. He meant it in a clinical sense, but I knew I was not ready for surgery psychologically. I had not yet reached the decision to proceed. I just wanted to know how I was going to reach that decision. About six months after I started asking him when I should have the surgery, I was ready. I knew it, and David knew it.

Surgery is sensible when your condition begins to interfere with the quality of life or when it substantially impairs the quality of life.

What happened during those six months? How did I change from being frustrated at the ambiguity in these phrases about substantial impairment of quality of life to knowing that I satisfied them? I cannot give you a completely definite response, but I can describe the process that I went through to reach that conclusion.

When I first began talking to David about hip surgery, my arthritis was a serious annoyance, but I could still get around easily enough. I was working out, strenuously swimming and weightlifting. I was aware of my condition sporadically throughout the day, but it had not yet become the brooding omnipresence it would develop into later. If I walked too far, I would be sore the next day, but gentle stretching and exercise would loosen my muscles up a bit. I still responded well to aspirin and naproxen. In general, if I was sensible in my activities—that is, exercising properly and stretching and taking pain medications—I could go about my business with only occasional serious discomfort.

Over the next six months, my condition changed dramatically. The pain level slightly but steadily increased. The joint became stiffer and stiffer and less responsive to stretching exercises, and I began having trouble sleeping. These were mild problems at first but more severe ones toward the end. Over the last eight weeks before surgery on my left hip, I had to fall asleep in between waves of pain. I would position myself comfortably and hope to fall asleep, because I knew that within five minutes I would suffer intense pain again. When that happened, I would reposition myself and try to sleep again. If I walked more than a few blocks, I would have a sharp pain in my hip that felt like I was walking on a spike. In fact, I could barely walk in a straight line. I essentially fell over my left hip and then strode on my right leg. Even when I was not experiencing serious, sharp pain, I was in discomfort, which ranged from barely perceptible pain to throbbing in the joint.

As these physical changes were occurring, my outlook on life began to change. My condition came to dominate my life. I was constantly aware that something was wrong, and constantly apprehensive of experiencing shooting pains in my hip. Everything that I did, I did with my arthritis in mind. I would decide to go to social events based on how comfortable I thought I would be. As time went on I went to fewer and fewer, not only because of the discomfort but also because of the increasingly powerful sense that everything in my life had become a chore. My previous ability to live with and accommodate my arthritis had changed; my outlook on life bordered on depression. Even going to a cocktail party could turn into a disaster. There might be no place for me to sit, or if there was a place and I sat down, I might not be able to get up. At work, I never knew if, when I was standing in front of one of my classes giving a lecture, I would have a spasm of pain so intense it would make me gasp.

After a few months of living with my ever-increasing discomfort, I began to feel I could not live that way much longer. I was not just becoming crippled; constant pain was becoming a part of my existence. No longer did the fact that the technology of artificial hips was continually improving have any persuasive force over me. Perhaps, if I had known that a breakthrough in hip replacements had been six months to a year away, I might have tried to tough it out, but with no more than incremental technological improvements on the horizon, I no longer considered this factor. Finally, I had come to recognize that the quality of my life had been substantially impaired, and it was time to act. The books and David, I can now say apologetically, were right. You reach a point at which you simply can't go on any longer, and that's the point when you should consider joint replacement surgery.

Should you wait to have surgery until you are living a life of agony? That is difficult to say, because the point at which the potential benefits from surgery outweigh the potential risks will differ for each person. Also, your own views about it will change over time as mine did. I put off surgery on my left hip for as long as possible. Had I waited much longer, I would have been forced to

FIGURE 4-3
Ron's Left Hip

A. *Pre-surgery: In 1988 Ron's x-rays showed evidence of severe arthritis in his left hip, which was very painful. X-rays of his right hip also showed moderately severe arthritis, but he felt little pain in his right hip.*

B. *Post-surgery: A few months after his left hip replacement, Ron resumed most normal activities. X-rays show a well-fixed, uncemented hip replacement.*

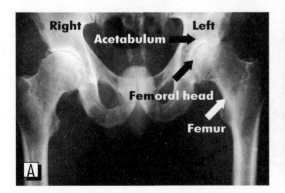

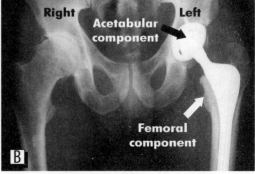

use a cane just to walk with acceptable levels of discomfort. I had quit playing tennis more than a year and half before the operation because the pain was too intense. (See Figure 4-3.)

Following my first surgery and the reasonably successful rehabilitation of my left hip, I concluded that I had waited too long to have the left hip replaced. I was not going to wait as long to operate on my right hip. I could not see any adequate reason to suffer as much as I did for as long as I did, given what I now knew about the options. This put me in conflict with David, whose view was, for good reason, that the decision to have surgery has to be made very cautiously. I did not disagree with that, but my view of acceptable levels of caution had come to differ somewhat from David's as a result of my experience with the surgery and its aftermath.

How Did I Decide to Replace My Right Hip?

OUR POTENTIAL DISAGREEMENT about how soon to operate on the right hip never occurred, however, because my right hip deteriorated much more rapidly than my left. In the course of about four months, I went from being reasonably comfortable, even after moderately intense tennis, to being unable to walk for more than five minutes on a flat surface without having the right hip feel like a vise grip had clamped down on it. The deterioration happened so quickly that I had only given up playing tennis about three weeks prior to the operation, although the last month of playing tennis was very difficult. (See Figure 4-4.)

FIGURE 4-4
Ron's Right Hip, Pre-Surgery

In 1993 Ron was having severe pain in his right hip. Although his left hip was quite comfortable, x-rays showed evidence of changes around his hip implant that suggested the plastic was wearing.

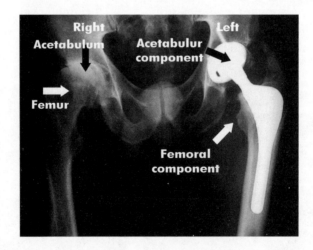

I TELL THIS ADDITIONAL STORY about my right hip because it emphasizes how difficult deciding when to have surgery is and how complex the variables are. One difference between my two primary surgeries is that I had been able to be more active on my right hip immediately before surgery than I had been before the operation on my left hip. As I mentioned, I had given up tennis a year and a half before the first operation and only a few weeks prior to the second. I had also been able to perform a rigorous strengthening program on my hips before the second operation that I had not done before the first one. For these reasons, the muscles in my right leg were in considerably better shape prior to the surgery than were the muscles in my left, resulting in an astounding difference in my rehabilitation. After the first surgery, I was walking without support in about six weeks; following the second surgery, it took only four. Moreover, I had considerable pain in my left hip for about six months following surgery; after six weeks, I had none in my right hip. I believe that most of this had to do with the fact that my right hip had not deteriorated nearly as much as my left prior to surgery.

ONE FACTOR IN THE BALANCE of risks and benefits is the difficulty and likely success of rehabilitation. The longer you wait to have surgery, the greater the probability of your muscles deteriorating, which will make the post-surgical rehabilitation more painful and more difficult. I believe that one true indication that surgery is appropriate is when you reach the point at which you can no longer maintain the strength in your muscles with an appropriate exercise regimen. When that becomes impossible, you have good reason to think about proceeding with surgery, even if you are not yet in agony. Of course, you may still wish to hold off, but in my view, when deciding whether to undergo surgery, too much emphasis is placed on the current state of discomfort, and too little is placed on the future discomfort that will come as withered muscles are rebuilt. Also, if your muscles are so weak that the discomfort in rebuilding their strength overwhelms your will to improve them, you will be limited forever in what you can do and how comfortable you are.

In addition, you cannot overlook the fact that hip surgery is major surgery, and problems can occur during major surgery.

How Did the Two Surgeries Differ?

How Did I Balance the Risks and Benefits of Surgery?

During both my operations, I was under a general anesthetic for more than five hours. General anesthetics are not risk-free, and the risks include such serious matters as brain damage and death. Therefore, I must emphasize that my assessment of the risk I am willing to take is purely personal. No one should encourage another to have major elective surgery, because it is a purely personal decision; one with life and death implications. No one can instruct you on such matters.

Selecting a Surgeon

THE PROCEDURE OF SELECTING a surgeon, and an accompanying team of doctors and therapists, is not easily reducible to a set of simple rules. We refer to the entire team here because anyone contemplating surgery needs to have in place a team of medical professionals, not just an orthopedic surgeon. The members of your team need to work together for you. You will need to have the close cooperation of your internist or family doctor and the active engagement of a physiatrist or physical therapist. If you have any other significant medical problems—diabetes, for instance—you also will need to have a relevant specialist engaged. Serious questions concerning anesthesiology will need to be resolved, and you will need to obtain advice that you trust. So it's important to conceptualize what the undertaking will involve.

What you need most to put a team together is knowledge. You need to know a fair amount about the various medical options that are available, as well as the medical preferences and ways of interacting—that is, the bedside manner—of the doctors available to assist you. Most importantly, you need to remember that you will be putting together a team of individuals to accomplish what *you* want done. That means you have to understand the medical options that are available to you and at least have a preliminary idea of what your objectives are.

To find a doctor you are comfortable with, consult widely to get references. Medical referral agencies, your family doctor, and your friends and colleagues should be able to help. With each surgeon's name you are given, probe the source for all the information you can get. What are the doctor's qualifications? Why does the source recommend that doctor? What is it about that doctor that your source commends? What is the doctor's experience? How many of these surgeries does the doctor perform each year? Is the doctor abreast of all the most recent techniques and materials? Why or why not? Whom does your source know who has had success with the doctor, and can you call that person?

Sources for Referral

A number of organizations can direct you to experienced hospitals and surgeons in your area. In particular, the American Academy of Orthopaedic Surgery, the Hip Society, and the Knee Society can provide you with names of surgeons and hospitals you may wish to consider. They can also send you literature that will help prepare you for your visit to the surgeon's office. The advantage of these sources of information is that they are relatively unbiased. These national organizations have no particular local or regional biases. Their primary goal is to assure that you have a successful surgical experience.

National Referral Organizations

If you have a preference for a specific hospital (perhaps your internist practices there) and wish to learn which orthopedic surgeons at that hospital are most experienced in joint replacement surgery, you might call the physician referral service which is often offered by the hospital. Although this resource will be somewhat more biased than the national organizations (the hospital wants to encourage you to go there for your joint replacement), these referral services are also interested in having your surgery at the hospital be successful. The referral service should know which orthopedic surgeons are most experienced in joint replacement surgery and should encourage you to consult them.

Local Referral Services

Your personal physician is also a potentially good resource for names of surgeons. Ask for the names of orthopedic

Your Personal Physician

surgeons experienced in joint replacement surgery. Your personal physician may also be able to provide you with useful information about the non-technical characteristics of surgeons that have been recommended to you. Because your physician knows you, he or she is perhaps in the best position to direct you to someone with whom you are likely to be comfortable.

If your physician knows or has worked with a particular orthopedic surgeon who is experienced in joint replacement surgery, you might ask him or her to contact that surgeon prior to your visit. Surgeons, like all conscientious service providers, are anxious to maintain a good relationship with their referral sources, including your physician, and thus will be responsive to his or her request for a prompt consultation. Moreover, your physician can provide the prospective surgeon with information about your health that will greatly assist him or her in your evaluation for surgery.

Friends and Former Patients

Friends and patients who have undergone joint replacement surgery are by far the most common source of referral to joint replacement surgeons. You will be surprised how many people have either undergone or know individuals who have undergone total joint replacement surgery, once you begin inquiring about total joint surgeons. If these friends or patients have had a positive experience with joint replacement surgery, they will enthusiastically recommend the procedure and, probably, the surgeon who performed them. These friends and patients can be important sources of support and encouragement. They can often describe what it is like to undergo replacement surgery and tell you what to expect. If, however, these friends or patients have had an unsuccessful or unhappy experience, they may discourage you from undergoing a procedure or consulting a specific surgeon. Thus, it is a good idea to balance the information from friends and patients, which is given with the best of intentions, with information that you have received from the other sources we have discussed.

Insurance Provider

Perhaps the referral source that is rapidly becoming the most frequently used by patients, voluntarily or not, is the insurance provider. You may belong to an insurance plan that specifies the orthopedic resources that you must use for your joint replacement. Virtually all insurance providers maintain a list of orthopedic surgeons covered by your plan. However, these providers have almost never specifically determined or stipulated that the list includes surgeons experienced in joint replacement surgery. Moreover, the provider may not be able to tell you which of its orthopedic surgeons is experienced in joint replacement surgery. Therefore, you may need to use the resources discussed above to obtain names of experienced joint replacement surgeons practicing at hospitals serviced by your insurance plan. If the list of surgeons provided by your plan does not include any names provided by such sources as the American Academy of Orthopaedic Surgeons, the Hip Society, or the Knee Society, you may need to include a visit to a surgeon from one of those sources at your own expense.

IN MANY WAYS, SELECTING A SURGEON may be more difficult than you think. Even physicians and surgeons who work closely with another surgeon have surprisingly little specific information regarding how competent that surgeon really is. Only an experienced surgeon who has actually observed and assisted another surgeon in his or her same field can accurately assess the competence of that surgeon. How then can you determine which surgeon is best suited to carry out your hip or knee replacement?

You should begin by determining how experienced a surgeon and the hospital at which he or she works are with joint replacement surgery. Joint replacement surgery is a team effort. It is most likely that you will have a competent team—including primary care physician, surgeon, anesthesiologist, therapists, nursing staff, and support staff—if your surgery is performed at a medical facility that carries out a significant number of joint replacements a year.

Results from a number of studies indicate that surgeons who frequently perform total joint replacements have better

The Surgeon's Experience

Determine how experienced a surgeon and the hospital are with joint replacement surgery.

results with fewer complications than do surgeons who only occasionally perform these procedures. Although it is not really possible to establish the minimum number of total joint replacements that should be done each year by a surgeon to ensure adequate familiarity with the procedures, experienced joint replacement surgeons usually do at least fifty such procedures a year.

Keep in mind that total hip replacement operations require different skills and experience than total knee replacement procedures. Some surgeons may be significantly more experienced with one or the other of the procedures. Inquire specifically about the surgeon's and the hospital's experience with the procedure you are to undergo.

Interviewing Surgeons

ONCE YOU HAVE NARROWED YOUR LIST to a few names, make an appointment to see each of the surgeons to discuss your situation. Take this opportunity to learn as much as you can about each doctor. Remember that you are the customer, and that ultimately you are responsible for your own care. Take a long list of questions about how the surgeon's standard procedures might help your particular problem. (See Table 4-1.) You are not just going for advice and assistance; you are deciding whether this person is going to perform major surgery on you. You have the right to probe what he or she has to say, and you should be satisfied with the answers on two levels: you should come away convinced that this person has complete command of the situation; and you should be convinced that you can work well with this person and that he or she is attuned to your concerns and willing to spend the time necessary to explain things to you.

What Should You Look for in the Surgeon?

Without a doubt the most important characteristic for you to try to identify, if possible, is whether the surgeon is honest: with you, with him- or herself, with your condition, and with the surgery and what it entails. Above all, you should have the feeling that the surgeon wants to do what is best for you. Although you may think that your visit to the surgeon is to discuss total joint surgery, the orthopedist

TABLE 4-1: Basic Questions to Ask the Surgeon

❏ The surgeon's background and experience
- Did you do a post-residency fellowship in total joint surgery or arthritis surgery?
- How many total joint replacements have you performed? How many total hips? How many total knees? Do you do total joint revision surgery?
- How long have you used the total joint implant system that will be used in my case? Why do you use it? Why is it appropriate for me?
- What are your biggest worries about total joint replacements? How do they apply to me?

❏ Outcomes of the surgeon's operations
- What are your results of the operation you are recommending? How do you know? Do you keep a record of your patients' outcomes?
- What are the most frequent complications? How do you try to keep these from happening?
- What are your patients' most common complaints about the surgery you are recommending that I undergo?

❏ Patient-surgeon communications
- How do I communicate with you before and after surgery? To whom do I address my questions? If I have an emergency, how do I reach you?
- How often do I see you after the proposed operation?

❏ Recommendations for the patient
- What is the best overall treatment program for me at this time?
- What would be the consequences of my not having total surgery now?
- If I decide to postpone total joint surgery, what should my activities be? What exercises should I do? What activities should I avoid?
- What activities do you allow or recommend after my proposed surgery?
- How long is my joint replacement likely to last?
- How successful is a revision of my joint replacement likely to be, if I need one? How long will that revision last?

❏ Hospital and staff capabilities
- How many total joint replacements are performed at the hospital where I would have my surgery?
- Are the assistants in the operating room specialists in orthopedics or joint replacement surgery?
- Does the hospital unit where I will receive my post-operative care specialize in orthopedics?
- What will my post-hospital discharge care be like?

Table 4-1, continued

❏ Physical therapy
 • How is physical therapy provided during my hospital stay?
 • Do I need pre-operative physical therapy?
 • Do you really think physical therapy is important after a total joint replacement?

❏ References
 • What are the names of surgeons that you would recommend as good sources of second opinions? If you needed the surgery that I am considering, whom would you have perform it?
 • Would you give me the names of patients similar to me on whom you have performed the type of surgery that you are recommending?

❏ Insurance
 • Will your charges for the procedure be completely covered by my insurance? Will my hospital charges be covered by insurance? How much will I have to pay out-of-pocket?

should be trying to determine what treatment, perhaps including surgery, is most appropriate for you now and in the future. *A significant proportion of patients referred to us for surgery not only do not need surgery at that moment but also may never require surgery!*

If you get the impression that the surgeon you are interviewing is not forthcoming or seems uninterested in spending substantial time with you, then leave. No matter how highly recommended someone is, you don't want him or her operating on you unless you are convinced that you will have his or her complete attention, that this person will treat you as the individual you are and respond to your individualized needs. Given the significance of what you are about to undergo, you should expect no less. And remember, you are probably entering into a long-term relationship with the person; it is clearly not too much to ask that such a relationship be built on a firm foundation.

What Should the Surgeon Do in the Interview?

The surgeon that you visit should listen to the history of your problem, examine you, review your previous treatment records and x-rays, evaluate your current x-rays, and explain to you the nature and current status of your hip or knee problem. He or she should explain the natural history of your situation and how various treatment approaches will affect that natural history. You should not feel as though there is a great urgency about your condition. With relatively rare exceptions, arthritis of the hip or knee is not a disease that requires emergency treatment. You should have the sense that you really have a choice in your treatment options. You should have the feeling that the orthopedist is as interested in being sure that you have the best non-surgical care as he or she is in providing the best surgical care.

As you inquire about the surgeon's experience, you should try to get a sense of how he or she interacts with all of the other providers that will take part in your care. You should feel that there will be in place a plan for your complete care, from the moment the surgery is scheduled until the point that you will no longer need his or her services, except for routine follow-up. Although your actions can very much influence the outcome of your surgery, it is the responsibility of the surgeon to make it possible for you to optimize your actions. The surgeon, his or her colleagues, the staff, and the hospital should facilitate your participation in the process of undergoing a total joint replacement.

How Does the Surgeon Interact with Team Members?

An issue of particular concern to patients is the availability of their surgeon if questions or problems arise before, during, or after the surgery. The best joint replacement surgeons, like the best of anything, are often the busiest. Nevertheless, experienced, high-quality surgeons recognize the importance of having experienced, competent personnel available at all times. It is important that you understand how you will communicate with your surgeon.

Some orthopedists share calls with their partners. If this is the case, you should determine the experience of the surgeon's partners with issues related to joint replacement surgery. Some surgeons have specially trained physician assistants or non-surgical musculoskeletal experts (such as physiatrists or rheumatologists) who are available to answer questions about your surgery. Many physicians have a combination of these two approaches.

It is important that you be comfortable with the communication system used by your surgeon. Many patients feel abandoned by their surgeon, especially after surgery. Surgeons are as interested as their patients in ensuring that this feeling of abandonment does not occur; this feeling is often the result of a lack of clear understanding from the start of the patient-surgeon relationship about the nature of the communication process used. Your prospective surgeon should be comfortable in discussing how he or she and the office communicate with patients before, during, and after surgery.

What Information Should the Surgeon Provide?

The surgeon, his or her staff, and the hospital should be able to provide you with a substantial amount of information about total joint surgery. They should be interested in doing so. The days when a surgeon could get away with simply proclaiming that a patient should leave the details of surgery and information about those details to him have long passed. If the questions you ask about the surgery are so technical that, in fact, you cannot understand the scientific explanation required, the orthopedist should explain the issue in a way that satisfies you that he or she is being as honest and complete as information about the issue allows.

The surgeon should also be able to describe his or her results with the procedure you are contemplating. It is fair and appropriate to ask what complications the surgeon has had, how often they have occurred, and what the surgeon does to minimize these complications. The surgeon may not be able to quote to you the exact results of his or her total joint surgery experience. However, the surgeon's approach to your request for information about these results is important to assess. All surgeons have complications. Experienced, mature surgeons acknowledge this fact and understand how they are trying to minimize them.

Which Patients Should the Surgeon Use as References?

You may find it helpful to talk to patients who have undergone a total joint replacement performed by the surgeon you are contemplating using. Ask the surgeon if you can talk with patients that have problems similar to yours. If you are young, if you are very active, if you are overweight, if you have a peculiar type of arthritis, if you have specific goals for your surgery, be sure that you speak to patients who are like you with regard to these issues. A surgeon's willingness and ability to identify patients with interests and goals similar to yours is a measure of that surgeon's awareness of and interest in you as a person with personally felt needs.

Would You Feel Safe in the Surgeon's Hands?

Perhaps the question that may be hardest to consider about your surgeon is the one that is most important. If you have a complication, perhaps a serious complication, would you feel safe and well cared for by the surgeon that you are considering? Neither you nor your prospective surgeon anticipate that you will have such a complication. The chances, in fact, are that you will go through your total joint surgery without a problem. However, it is likely that little hitches will occur along the way (for instance, the blood bank might not be able to draw your blood or the post-operative therapist may be late in starting). It is much less likely, but possible, that you will have a more serious complication. You must be as sure as possible that the surgeon, his or her staff, and the physicians, health professionals, and hospital are capable of and comfortable with dealing with such unwanted outcomes. The true measure of a good joint replacement surgeon is his or her ability to deal effectively and compassionately with an unexpected or undesired result.

Seeking a Second, or Even a Third, Opinion

BECAUSE THE SELECTION of an appropriate surgeon is critical to the ultimate success of your joint replacement procedure, it is important that you be as comfortable as possible with your ultimate selection. We recommend that you plan to visit at least two surgeons before making your selection. Even if the first surgeon that you visit has all of the qualifications that you want (including proper references, appropriate experience, desirable personality), a visit to a second or third surgeon can be useful. You will invariably receive additional information about joint replacement surgery.

Usually, the second surgeon will reinforce the opinion of the first and you will find this reassuring. If the opinions differ widely, then you probably need to keep seeking information. Do not be embarrassed to ask a surgeon whom he or she would recommend to give a second opinion! Experienced, mature joint replacement surgeons know that it is important for you to become as well informed about and comfortable with the surgery as possible. These surgeons will and should encourage you to obtain second or third opinions.

A Patient's Perspective: Ron

WHEN I FIRST MET DAVID, what struck me most was his willingness to discuss things. As we progressed toward the first surgery, I spent more and more time in the medical library learning about my condition, treatment options, and new research that was being performed. When I met with David, I had a long list of questions, which he took the time to go through with me. I became convinced that his reputation was justified. He obviously had a complete command of his field, and his explanations were sensible. As impressed with his technical prowess as I was, I was equally impressed with his candor. He did not act defensively or impatiently to my many questions, but dealt with them all in a calm and supportive fashion. He was not trying to dictate an approach, but was instead explaining the options that were available.

Selecting the Implant

A GREAT DEAL OF EFFORT has been spent since the 1970s to develop total joint implants that allow high levels of activity and last a long time. It is, therefore, appropriate and important for you to be familiar with implant issues that could affect both the immediate and long-term function of your joint replacement. You can become knowledgeable about many of the characteristics of the devices that will be used to replace your hip or knee. This information will help you discuss more intelligently your upcoming surgery with your surgeon. It will also help you understand how various implant choices might affect your post-operative recovery.

IT IS VERY IMPORTANT when thinking about total joint implant issues to keep in mind three facts:

Joint Implant Issues

❏ The *way* total joint implants are inserted is much more likely to influence their quality and longevity than is any specific design characteristic.

❏ Many implants currently available are very likely to last fifteen to twenty years or more.

❏ Many total hip and total knee replacement devices give essentially equivalent results.

Thus, the first and most important step you should take to make sure you will receive implants that function well and last a long time is to select a competent, experienced surgeon. Second, recognize that there is a very strong urge within all of us, patients and physicians, to want the latest in technology. However, some or perhaps many of the new implants and surgical techniques that are being or will be investigated may not prove over time to be improvements over what is currently available. The vast majority of patients, including relatively young (from fifty to sixty-five years old) and very active patients, will be best served by implants that have established a successful track record since the mid-1980s.

The patients who will benefit most from new technologies under current or future evaluation have one or more of the following characteristics:

❏ They are very young, less than fifty years of age.

❏ They are unusual or unique with regard to their musculoskeletal anatomy, such as having a developmental abnormality.

❏ They require a revision of their current total joint implant.

This last point needs clarification. Although primary (first-time) total joint implants are likely to last twenty years or more, prostheses used for revision (replacement) implants historically have lasted a much shorter period of time. Thus, patients undergoing revision surgery should make a particular effort to become informed about recent developments in total joint implant technology.

Ron's experience illustrates all of the issues that we have just been talking about. At the time that he needed his first—that is, his left—hip replacement, he was very young and physically active. In addition, he had a type of developmental hip abnormality that made it more difficult to use then-available implants. Thus, Ron was the type of patient for whom new technological developments are most appropriate. After much thought and discussion, Ron and we chose to use a custom, uncemented femoral hip implant and an uncemented acetabular prosthesis.

Although these devices functioned well for many years, they have ultimately needed to be revised. When Ron had his right hip replaced, just a few years after his left hip replacement, the technology for producing custom, uncemented implants had improved to the point that Ron felt the difference from the start. Evidence in his right hip of wear and loosening of the implant, which eventually led to the revision of his left hip, has not yet occurred, though Ron has been extremely active since that second hip surgery.

Moreover, when Ron required a revision of his first (left) hip replacement, he was still very young and active. He, again, was the type of patient for whom new technological developments are most appropriate. We therefore evaluated the new implant and bone grafting technologies that might best meet his needs. We selected devices and techniques that, though they had not yet been available for many years, seemed to be most appropriate for Ron's specific needs. His experience illustrates the benefits and, perhaps, the drawbacks of being the recipient of new total joint technology.

Therefore, the first question you should ask the surgeon that you have decided upon is, How many years has a given implant been used? A closely related and even more important question is, How long have you, the surgeon, been using a given implant? It is appropriate and helpful to your understanding of the procedure for you to ask your surgeon to explain why he or she uses whatever implant system is being selected for you. Table 4-2 lists these and other questions you should ask about the implants that you and your surgeon are considering. Table 4-3 provides some guidelines to help you decide how suitable the surgeon's response is to your question about why a particular implant is most appropriate for you.

TABLE 4-2: Basic Questions to Ask About the Implant

❑ History and type of implant
  • How many years has the type of implant I will receive been used?
  • Is the implant I will receive cemented or uncemented? Why?
  • What issues of wear have arisen with this implant?
  • Do other surgeons at the hospital or in the region use this implant?

❑ Surgeon's experience with the implant
  • How long have you been using this type of implant?
  • Have you taken special courses on the use of the implant that I will receive? How did you learn to use it?

❑ Implant issues related to the patient
  • Is there anything about my particular situation that would make this implant inappropriate?
  • Are there new developments in joint replacement surgery that I should be aware of? Is it worth my while to wait for these developments to become available?

TABLE 4-3:
Why Has the Surgeon Selected a Particular Implant?

❑ Acceptable responses
  • The track record of the implant
  • The personal experience over a number of years with the device
  • The specific characteristics of the prosthesis that are likely to be helpful in your case, especially if the device has been in use a relatively short time

❑ Unacceptable responses
  • The cost of the implant
  • The availability at the specific hospital where the surgery is to be performed
  • The current popularity of the theory behind the design of the prosthesis

Possible Conflicts of Interest in Implant Selection

IF THE SURGEON THAT YOU HAVE SELECTED performs a large number of joint replacements or works at an institution known for joint replacement surgery, it is possible that he or she is involved in the development or clinical evaluation of new implant systems. On the one hand, this may be advantageous to you, for the surgeon may have access to and experience with devices that are not commonly available. On the other hand, the surgeon or surgeon's institution may, appropriately and legally, be receiving something of value for the development or evaluation work that he or she is carrying out in relation to the implants that are to be used in you. For instance, the surgeon may receive a consultation fee for working with the company that produces the implants, or the hospital or university at which the surgeon works may receive research support for participation in the development or evaluation work being performed. Your surgeon is obligated, ethically if not legally, to make you aware of the institution's or his or her involvement in this work.

Issues of Fixation

THERE ARE TWO IMPORTANT ASPECTS of fixation: the rigidity of the initial fixation and the longevity of that fixation. Complete pain relief can occur after total joint surgery only if the implants are rigidly fixed to bone. Pain relief will be sustained over the years only if the implants remain rigidly fixed.

Total joint implants are fixed to bone either with bone cement or by a process known as biological fixation. There are five issues about these means of fixation that are helpful to know.

First, both types of fixation, cemented and biological fixation, have proved to be virtually equally effective if correctly applied. Original concerns about the use of cement in younger, more active, heavier patients have decreased dramatically as the techniques for inserting cement and the quality of the cements have improved. Thus, many surgeons are comfortable inserting cemented total hip and knee implants in active, larger patients who are forty or fifty years of age. There are data to support this approach. Yet many surgeons feel that it is desirable to insert biologically fixed implants in older, smaller, less active patients—that is, those normally felt to be ideal for cemented devices. Substantial data also support this approach.

Second, total knee implants are much more likely than total hip replacements to be fixed with bone cement than with biological fixation, regardless of a patient's age, size, or level of activity. Many studies have shown that the fixation of cemented total knee implants is superior to, longer lasting than, and more reliable than the fixation obtained using the biological approach.

Third, some total joint implants are more easily and reliably fixed with cement and others with biological fixation. For example, the acetabular component of a total hip replacement can be most reliably fixed with biological fixation, while the femoral component can be most reliably fixed with cement. Thus, your surgeon may indicate that he or she will use a combination of cement and biological fixation to secure your implants to bone. This is called a hybrid fixation and is very commonly used in total hip surgery.

Fourth, it may be necessary to decide the method of fixation of the implants at the time of surgery. Factors that affect the selection of fixation, such as shape of the bone or quality of the bone, often cannot be precisely determined until it is examined during surgery. Thus, your surgeon may explain that while he or she usually uses one type of fixation, the final decision about the means of fixation in your case may not be made until the bone is being prepared for insertion of the implant.

Fifth, cemented implants in general cost less than uncemented implants. If a hospital is receiving a fixed reimbursement from your insurance carrier for your total joint replacement, it will attempt to reduce the costs of that replacement in a number of ways. Implant costs represent a significant portion of the total cost of the hospital's expense. Thus, because hospitals vigorously attempt to control implant costs, they may discourage the use of the more costly uncemented implants if reimbursement is fixed.

Thus, Medicare patients—patients age sixty-five or older—routinely receive cemented implants. Reported results with cemented implants in patients over the age of sixty-five have been very good. If you are older than sixty-five and receive a cemented replacement, the likelihood that it will remain well fixed for the rest of your life is very high. However, if you are over sixty-five and are very active or very large and believe that there might be an advantage to using a biologically fixed device in your case, you should discuss this with your surgeon.

Fixation and the Type of Implant

Ron received a custom femoral component for both of his replacements. Why? Because he was unusually young and very active, we decided to use implants that would become biologically fixed—that is, uncemented.

It is possible to design femoral implants that fit into the bone exactly. This is done by obtaining a computerized scan of the bone and building a computer model of the bone from that scan. A custom implant can then be designed and made which optimally fits within that bone. Because we have been involved for many years in the development of custom implant technology and explained its application in Ron's case, we decided with Ron that a custom, biologically fixed implant would be most appropriate for his situation.

Many surgeons who perform uncemented total hip replacements feel that custom implants are unnecessary. They believe that they can achieve an excellent long-term result using so-called off-the-shelf devices. These implants are made in many different sizes and shapes to fit a wide variety of bone conditions. Surgeons choose a system of off-the-shelf devices that they feel best meet the needs of patients undergoing uncemented total hip replacements. Surgeons then select the size of implant in that system they think most appropriate for a specific case.

Surgeons who use off-the-shelf implants do not feel that the extra cost of custom implants (approximately $1000 at the time Ron had his replacements) is justified by the results. Those of us who are proponents of custom femoral hip replacements believe that the reliability of fit, the quality of fixation achieved, and the quality of bone response to the custom implants more than justifies, especially over time, the additional cost.

Fixation and the Implants Used in Revision Surgery

Fixation issues in revision joint replacement surgery are more complex than those in primary surgery. In revision surgery the amount of bone available on which to place implants is reduced, often markedly, and the quality of bone is often poor. Thus, special implants may be necessary to achieve secure, long-lasting fixation and a combination of fixation techniques may be required. If you are about to undergo revision surgery, it is more important for you to determine the experience and expertise of your surgeon and his or her institution than for you to determine which type of implant and fixation technique should be used. In revision surgery, the surgeon and hospital must have a variety of implants and fixation methods available and they must be experienced in their use.

Durability

THE DURABILITY OF THE MATERIALS, especially the plastic, used in total joint implants is probably the most important factor affecting the longevity of the replacements. There is no doubt that the materials used today are more durable than they were in the 1980s. The plastics (polyethylenes) are much more consistent in quality. The finishes on the metals that work with the plastics are much finer. The methods for securing the plastics to metal are superior to those of a few years ago. Nevertheless, many issues about implant durability are incompletely understood.

You should ask questions of your surgeon about this important issue: How does he or she deal with the issue of implant durability? Does he or she use implants with a track record of longevity? Does he or she feel that you have special concerns with regard to this issue? How long does he or she feel a total joint implant is likely to last in your case and why? Are there things that you can do to increase the longevity of the implant? For example, there is information emerging that if osteoporosis is corrected in patients with total joint implants, the fixation of the implants may be more secure *and* the consequences of material wear, if it occurs, will be less severe. Thus, your surgeon may wish to determine if you are osteoporotic and treat this condition.

Total joint implants should remain well-fixed and durable for fifteen to twenty years.

Remember, most total joint implants used today should remain *well-fixed* and *durable* for fifteen to twenty years, if properly inserted. Therefore, perhaps the most important question that you can ask your surgeon about the implants to be used is this: Is there a reason why the selected implant may not last fifteen to twenty years? If there is, then you may wish to determine if it is necessary to use special implants to increase the likelihood of improving their longevity. The use of the new technologies that are currently under development

and evaluation should be reserved for those circumstances where it is reasonable to believe that currently available, well-tested implant systems and surgical techniques will not last at least fifteen to twenty years. Remember, many total joint technologies developed since the 1970s and promoted as providing greater function and longevity resulted in *less* longevity and *poorer* function than implants in use at the time the new technologies were introduced.

BEFORE YOUR SURGERY, it is critical to plan for the post-operative treatment and rehabilitation necessary after you leave the hospital. Those patients who are moderately debilitated before surgery or who will not have someone to care for them at home after the surgery benefit most from a period of rehabilitation in an inpatient facility. This post-operative inpatient rehabilitation may occur either in a rehabilitation unit or a nursing home.

Just as surgeons differ, rehabilitation facilities vary widely. Most surgeons refer to facilities near their own hospital. Proximity to your surgeon is very important but not critical. While you are in rehabilitation, you may not see your surgeon unless problems arise.

You will want to make sure the rehabilitation facility you plan to use has three important features. *First, you will need to see a rehabilitation physician regularly*, and unless your surgeon recommends a particular physician or physiatrist, you may be assigned to the managing physiatrist at the facility. You should find out how frequently that physician performs rounds at the rehabilitation hospital. Physiatrists in traditional rehabilitation hospitals see their patients either every day or several days a week. However, many rehabilitation units in nursing homes do *not* have physicians who circulate that regularly. In these units you are more likely to see a physician once a week unless problems arise. We believe that you will receive better care if you have the opportunity to see a physician at least three times a week when you are in rehabilitation.

Second, you should choose only a facility that offers therapy on a daily basis, seven days a week. Many facilities do not offer therapy on Saturdays and Sundays. Those facilities are entirely *unacceptable* for joint replacement patients, who need to receive a *minimum* of two hours of physical therapy every day.

Third, the therapy and nursing care you receive in rehabilitation should follow protocols of care, which are well established for joint replacement patients. Complications from surgery can occur if therapy and nursing care are not performed accurately. The wound must be cared for diligently, splints or

Selecting an Inpatient Rehabilitation Unit

other devices need to be applied appropriately, and therapy must be performed according to the specific instructions of the surgeon. The rehabilitation physicians, nurses, and allied health staff must be able to identify quickly if your progress is not proceeding as expected. Minor interventions can often avert major catastrophes. Therefore, it is extremely important for your rehabilitation facility to have *expertise* in joint replacement care.

The Costs of Joint Replacement and Your Insurance Coverage

THE GOAL OF THE PATIENT, the patient's family, the physician, and the physician's office staff in the preoperative period is to prepare the patient physically, emotionally, and financially to achieve a successful joint replacement outcome. To achieve this goal, you need to know what the costs of total joint surgery are.

Costs

THE ACTUAL COST OF SURGERY is more of a factor for some people than is it for others. Currently, Medicare, Medicaid, and all private insurance companies, including health maintenance organizations (HMOs), cover the cost of surgery. HMOs and private provider organizations (PPOs), however, may restrict where the surgery is performed. Average charges for the acute care hospital stay for a total hip replacement are well over $30,000, slightly lower for a knee replacement procedure. Additional inpatient rehabilitation care adds about $14,000 to that price. Outpatient physical therapy averages another $2,500, and home health outpatient services, $2,000 to $4,000. These are charges, however, and not what it *costs* the hospital to care for you or what your insurance company *pays*. Most insurance companies pay only a portion of the bill they receive from hospitals. You may or may not be responsible for the balance of the bill, depending upon the limits of your coverage.

Determining Actual Coverage

ONCE YOU AND YOUR SURGEON have established the need for total joint replacement, you need to know how much your insurance will pay of the total costs of the procedure. Many resources exist to help you through the maze of insurance requirements related to total joint replacement surgery. *You need to clearly understand how much of the surgery and after-care is covered by your insurance, and what you will be expected to pay.* The first and probably most helpful source should be the surgeon and his or her office staff. Be aware that surgeons are required to obtain pre-certification from your insurance company before performing surgery. Because of this, your surgeon's office personnel who process the insurance paperwork should be very familiar with the issues related to coverage for the entire joint replacement process. You should feel comfortable seeking this information from your surgeon because he or she is in the best position to direct you to the most relevant and helpful information about insurance coverage.

In addition, consult your insurance company and the hospital for information about the extent of your insurance coverage for a total joint replacement. It may take many phone calls and letters to your insurance provider to get a straight answer, but be persistent. Remember to obtain as much information *in writing* as you can.

Obtain as much information in writing as you can.

There are also many social and community services that may be available to you both before and after surgery. You should ask your surgeon about the availability of these services and seek to obtain as many services as you need to ensure a successful outcome. Many of the services are paid for by various insurance programs.

Legal Liability and the Potential for Conflicts of Interest

Negligence and Malpractice

UNDERGOING JOINT REPLACEMENT SURGERY provides you with the potential to live a normal, pain-free life. However, there are risks associated with the surgery that you need to take into account. The presence of these risks affects your doctor's relationship with you. The threat of legal liability for malpractice lurks in the background of any medical treatment, and thus unavoidably affects the decision-making of doctors.

YOUR DOCTORS ARE LEGALLY LIABLE for any negligent mistakes that they make that cause you harm. Precisely just what constitutes a negligent mistake is complicated. Briefly, it is any treatment, or failure to treat, that falls below the general standards of the relevant medical field. However, merely because something does not work out perfectly does not mean a doctor is liable for what went wrong. Sometimes procedures just don't work out. Even if done perfectly, a procedure often has less than a one hundred percent chance for success. If in your case the doctor does everything correctly, but the operation still does not succeed, it is unfortunate, but there would be no liability. But if your doctor fails to do something that most other doctors under the same circumstances would have done, and his or her action causes you harm, then the doctor may be liable.

The reality of medical malpractice is more complex than this description of liability suggests. Often, what constitutes the standards in a field of medicine are unclear, and often the relevant facts, such as about the patient's symptoms, are unclear or disputed. Consequently, predicting what acts will lead to liability for malpractice is extremely difficult to do.

The ambiguity surrounding malpractice has a definite effect on the medical profession. It makes doctors cautious. To some extent, this is very good. It encourages doctors to take great care and pay close attention to what they are doing. In addition to inducing caution, the threat of liability also induces a certain conservatism in judgment. Doctors want to help you get well, but they also want to avoid liability to themselves.

TYPICALLY A DOCTOR'S DESIRE to help you and to avoid personal financial harm are not in conflict, but from time to time they are. This is especially true when the advice a doctor gives relates to procedures such as hip and knee surgery.

Only rarely would a doctor be found liable for malpractice for *not* recommending or performing a joint replacement surgery. Liability virtually always results from surgery gone awry. Thus, the risk of legal liability puts pressure on physicians to delay surgical intervention as long as possible in all cases that pose no risk in delay except for the patient's increased discomfort. The prospect of liability also encourages doctors to choose treatment alternatives that have fewer, less severe complications, even if a somewhat riskier alternative has a higher probability of providing more satisfactory results.

However, not all forces acting on doctors lead to conservative advice. Offsetting the pressure of legal liability that may lead an orthopedic surgeon to discourage you from having a joint replacement is the prospect for the surgeon of personal financial gain from doing the surgery. Surgeons will not be sued for advising against surgery, but their income will go down significantly if they perform only a few surgeries. Thus, this personal financial incentive could lead a surgeon to give overly aggressive advice about the need for surgery.

Your best preparation for dealing with these conflicting concerns of your surgeon is to be as informed as possible about your condition, its implications, and the true risks and benefits of the treatments available to you.

M OST DOCTORS DO THE BEST THEY CAN and truly have their patients' best interests uppermost in their minds. We do not want to even hint to the contrary. Our purpose here is quite different. It is to help you understand the very complex position doctors are in. That understanding should make you aware of your own responsibility in making decisions about your care and treatment. Educate yourself, ask

Possible Divergence of Interests Between You and Your Doctor

Conclusion

for full explanations from your doctors, and demand that you get them. Take responsibility for your own care: that is the single most important message of this book.

PREPARING
for SURGERY

THE TIME HAS FINALLY COME. You have learned about and learned to live with your arthritic hip or knee. But total joint replacement surgery is now inevitable for you, so you have gathered a lot of information about the procedure and the implants that are available. Most importantly, you have selected your surgeon and hospital to perform the replacement. You are sure that your decision to proceed with a total joint replacement is appropriate. You are ready, perhaps even anxious, to proceed. This chapter describes the preparations that you should now carry out for your joint surgery.

Pre-Operative Medical Evaluation

Preparing for a total joint replacement is, in many respects, no different from preparing for any major surgical procedure. You must, for example, obtain a careful medical evaluation to be sure that it is safe to proceed. This medical evaluation, done by your primary care physician, usually includes a thorough physical examination, a number of blood tests, an electrocardiogram, a chest x-ray, and a urinalysis.

Special tests may be necessary if you have certain risk factors. If you are a smoker or have lung disease, for instance, you may need to undergo pulmonary function tests. If you are at risk for heart disease, your physician may want you to undergo a cardiac stress test before surgery to make sure your heart is able to withstand the stress of the surgical procedure.

Many pre-operative issues—such as medication, precautions against infection, donating blood, nutrition, and physical conditioning—specifically influence total joint replacement, so you need to be aware of them.

Discontinuing Medication before Surgery

Almost all patients who have arthritis that is severe enough to require total joint replacement surgery take medication to control pain and inflammation. Many of these drugs, however, affect the normal ability of blood to clot, so you must stop using them at a specified time before surgery. If the anti-inflammatory drugs are not stopped prior to surgery, excessive bleeding from tissue that has been cut may occur during and after the operation. This excessive bleeding could also cause increased pain, decreased motion, and in extreme cases injury to nerves or muscles in the operated leg. Therefore, it is important that these tissues not have an increased tendency to bleed. Medications are available to help ease your discomfort in the interim, however.

THE LENGTH OF TIME it takes for the clotting effect to wear off varies with the medication. Aspirin and aspirin-containing products, for example, should be stopped ten to fourteen days before surgery. Nonsteroidal, anti-inflammatory medications, such as the once-a-day versions of Lodine, Voltaren, or Relafen, should be stopped seven days before surgery. Anti-inflammatory agents taken two to four times a day (ibuprofen, naproxen, or diclofenac) should be stopped two to four days before surgery. Acetaminophen-containing drugs, such as Tylenol, do not affect clotting and can be taken up to the day of surgery.

You may be taking other medications that affect blood clotting. You should ask your primary care physician about this. For example, if you have heart disease and take the blood thinner warfarin (Coumadin), you must stop taking it a number of days before your surgery. However, if you need to maintain the effects of warfarin until the day of the surgery, your physician may wish to substitute heparin, which has a shorter duration of effect.

To keep drugs from interfering with blood clotting, then, you must stop taking them far enough before your surgery to permit their effects to wear off. We can't emphasize this issue strongly enough. Be sure to discuss your medication schedule with your doctor weeks before the surgery.

MANY PEOPLE EXPERIENCE a significant increase in pain when they stop using their arthritis medications just before surgery. You should anticipate this and ask your physician for alternative pain medication, such as acetaminophen, codeine, or hydrocodone, that you can use in the interim. People with rheumatoid arthritis who take anti-rheumatic agents such as prednisone, methotrexate, and immuran can take these medicines up until the day of surgery. Your physician may, however, need to change the dosage of these medications immediately before or after surgery. You should discuss this with your primary care doctor well before your operation, and make sure the orthopedic team is aware of the medication changes.

The Anti-Clotting Effects of Specific Kinds of Medications

To keep drugs from interfering with blood clotting, you must stop taking them far enough before your surgery to permit their effects to wear off.

Interim Pain Medications

Precautions against Infection

THE MOST DEVASTATING orthopedic-related complication of total joint replacement surgery is infection around the prosthesis. Many precautions are taken before, during, and after surgery to prevent this from occurring. An important step in preparing for surgery is to establish that no source of infection exists. Total joint replacement surgery should be postponed if a source of infection is discovered in the pre-operative evaluation.

It is a good idea to have a dental examination a few weeks before your surgery. If a potential source of infection is found, there will be time to treat it before you undergo your replacement.

In your pre-operative medical exam you will be asked to give a urine sample to verify that you don't have a bladder infection. Because asymptomatic bladder infections are quite common in women, many surgeons request that all of their female patients take a short course of antibiotics before surgery. If the urine sample obtained before surgery reveals an infection, a more extended course of antibiotics may need to be taken prior to surgery. Men with a history of prostate disease should be particularly alert to the possibility of a urinary tract infection.

Donating Blood for Possible Transfusion

HIP AND KNEE REPLACEMENT SURGERY may result in the loss of a significant amount of blood. Many patients receive transfusions of one to two units of blood during or immediately after knee replacement surgery, and up to three units during or after hip replacement surgery. The safest way to be transfused is to receive your own blood. You can donate the required number of units in the weeks before your surgery. Your orthopedic surgeon and his or her staff can give you the details about participating in a blood donation program. Blood banks are available in nearly all towns. You can therefore arrange to donate the blood near your home and have it sent to the hospital, even if the hospital is a long distance from your home. If you cannot donate your own blood—

because you have heart disease or anemia, or because you take certain medications—you may be able to arrange for a close relative to donate his or her blood for you.

You are least likely to need a blood transfusion after surgery if your red blood cell count, usually expressed as grams-of-hemoglobin or hematocrit, is close to normal prior to surgery. A normal hemoglobin is between 13–15 grams, which is roughly equivalent to a hematocrit of 40–50. You can help ensure that your red blood cell count is as high as possible by taking iron supplements and by eating nutritionally well-balanced meals.

If you have a low blood count, you may benefit from a new medicine, erythropoietin. It has been approved for use before and immediately after joint replacement surgery to maximize your blood count and minimize the need for blood transfusion. This medication stimulates your body to produce blood. However, it requires weekly injections prior to surgery, and not all patients with low blood counts should take erythropoietin. Ask your doctor if you are a suitable candidate for this drug.

The Importance of Good Nutrition

GOOD NUTRITION IS VERY IMPORTANT before joint replacement surgery. Patients who are even slightly malnourished are more likely to develop infections and have problems with their surgical wounds healing than patients who are well nourished. Ask your physician to recommend a diet for the weeks before your surgery. Nutritional supplements may be useful for people who are very thin or who have low blood levels of body proteins. These supplements, such as Ensure, Sustacal, and Carnation Instant Breakfast, are available without a prescription.

Physical Condition- ing before Surgery

Y OU SHOULD TRY TO MAXIMIZE your physical condition before surgery. Being physically fit will make your post-operative recovery easier and shorter. Severe arthritis invariably leads to muscle weakness, stiffness, and reduced aerobic conditioning. Surgery itself also reduces strength, motion, and endurance. For example, key muscles, such as the quadriceps muscle at the knee or gluteus medius muscle of the hip, may lose more than half of their strength imme- diately after surgery. The stronger your muscles are going into surgery, the easier it will be to exercise and get around after surgery.

Sometimes pain from a bad hip or knee is so severe be- fore surgery that exercise seems impossible. Usually, however, most people can find ways to keep up strength and condition- ing despite this pain. One way is to exercise in a warm pool. The arthritis pool classes sponsored by the Arthritis Founda- tion are a nice way to exercise before surgery. The warmth and buoyancy of the water helps facilitate pain-free exercise. Also, a physiatrist or physical therapist can develop a modified home exercise program to help you maintain strength and endur- ance, in spite of your painful joint.

Planning for the Initial Weeks after Surgery

T OTAL JOINT REPLACEMENT SURGERY will have a significant effect on your life and the lives of those around you for the first few weeks after your discharge from the hospital. These weeks are the most critical to your rehabilitation. There- fore, it is very important that you and your family and friends prepare for this time. Your orthopedist and your hospital will also help with this preparation. Many medical centers provide a special pre-operative class for patients who plan to undergo hip or knee replacement. Some centers have representatives of the replacement team visit your home prior to surgery. These pre-operative programs help to inform you and your family about the procedure, optimize your arrangements at home for your recovery, and familiarize you with some of the early post- operation therapy techniques, such as walking with crutches.

Although your surgeon and his or her team will try to plan as accurately as possible for your post-discharge destination (whether to a rehabilitation facility or directly to your home), it is not unusual for those plans to change during your hospital stay. Your destination following your discharge from the hospital will be based on your post-surgical condition and your capacity to progress with your therapy.

IF YOU ARE OLDER or are, in general, less mobile, you may elect to transfer from the hospital to a rehabilitation unit. You will remain in the unit until you are able to care for yourself. This usually takes one to two weeks. Your hospital may have such a unit in or near the main acute care facility. Or, if the hospital is far from your home, you may want to select a rehabilitation facility closer to your home or family. Familiarize yourself with the inpatient rehabilitation options available to you before your surgery.

The Rehabilitation Facility

MANY SERVICES ARE AVAILABLE for those patients who go directly home from the hospital. For example, you may be able to have an attendant to help you bathe, a nurse to draw blood or help with surgical dressing changes, and physical and occupational therapists to help you regain your ability to function normally. Even if you are older and live alone, these services may be all that you need to go directly home after surgery. Discuss these issues with a social worker, nurse, or discharge planner at the hospital or at the doctor's office before your surgery so that appropriate plans can be made.

In-Home Care

BY THE TIME YOU ARE SENT HOME, you will be walking with crutches or a walker and basically will be able to care for yourself. However, preparing meals, doing laundry and housekeeping, carrying heavy objects, climbing stairs, or caring for someone else will be difficult for the first few weeks after surgery. Therefore, you may want to prepare and freeze some meals before surgery, arrange for grocery delivery for the first month after surgery, and use a cleaning service for your house

Daily Chores and Errands

or laundry. If you live alone, plan to have a friend or relative stay with you for a week or two to help you.

As you make your plans for recovering at home from your surgery, always keep in mind that the goal of joint replacement surgery is to restore you to the daily functions that you would be capable of with a normal hip or knee. Attaining this goal requires not only that your surgeon performs the surgical procedure properly, but also that you carry out your post-operative rehabilitation plan properly at home.

Assessing Your Health Insurance Coverage

PERHAPS ONE OF THE MOST IMPORTANT and occasionally the most frustrating pre-operative activity that you and your health care team must perform is a careful and accurate assessment of your health care insurance coverage for the proposed total joint replacement procedure and the post-discharge recovery period. As we discussed in Chapter 4, insurance coverage of the services for care for total joint replacement patients varies widely. Medicare and most private insurance plans currently do not place significant restrictions on the pre-operative evaluation that your surgeon and physician are likely to request, but they may change their policies soon, so be aware of this possibility. Unusual tests, such as CT scans, may not be covered. If you require unusual tests as part of your pre-operative evaluation, clarify who will pay for such tests before they are performed.

If you are asked by your physicians, including your anesthesiologist, to participate in a study, such as one for a new prosthesis, anesthetic agent, or blood clot preventive drug, be sure that the costs of any special tests required by the study are paid for by the sponsor, which is often a drug company.

Authorization for the Length of Stay at the Hospital

AUTHORIZATION FOR AN INPATIENT STAY beyond the specified number of days usually will be granted only after representatives of the insurance carrier have received additional details of your hospital stay from the hospital and surgeon's office staff. This requirement may place your health care providers in the difficult position of having to explain to you and your family why you cannot continue to stay in the hospital and receive the inpatient care you perceive would be helpful. You can avoid this annoyance if you are aware, before your admission, of the number of days of acute inpatient post-surgical care that your insurance carrier has certified.

INSURANCE AUTHORIZATION FOR INPATIENT CARE, while sometimes burdensome to obtain, usually results in complete coverage of the procedure and post-operative inpatient care. However, the insurance coverage for post-discharge care varies widely among carriers. The extent of your coverage will greatly influence the care you are likely to receive once you leave the hospital. For example, Medicare and most private insurers pay for post-discharge inpatient rehabilitation after a total joint replacement only for those patients who meet certain functional criteria, such as the need for basic self-care, or help with bed-to-chair transfers. In addition, insurance policies differ widely on the amount and type of at-home nursing and therapy services that patients are eligible to receive.

Coverage of Post-Discharge Care

It is important that you and your family understand the limits of your health care coverage before you have surgery so you can plan for your post-discharge care responsibly and realistically. If you are concerned that your coverage will not be adequate for your recovery, discuss these concerns with your surgeon and his or her staff. There are a number of legitimate ways to go "out of contract" and get services covered if the services can be established as medically necessary. You may need to ask your surgeon and primary care doctor to support in writing the medical necessity of post-operative services not routinely covered by your insurance plan. Persistence is the key to success in obtaining permission for such services. Finally, be sure authorization for the requested services is in writing.

Conclusion

ONCE PREPARATIONS FOR SURGERY are complete, you will be ready to undergo the procedure. Although you will be understandably nervous, you are also likely to be anxious to proceed. In fact, it is very common for patients to experience substantially more than the usual amount of pain in the affected joint in the few days prior to surgery. This may be the result of stopping your anti-inflammatory and analgesic medications or it may due to increasing tension. This tension will be easier to handle if you understand at least some of the details of the procedure you are about to undergo.

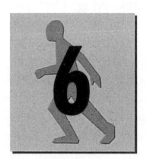

SURGERY

YOU ARE NOW ABOUT TO undergo a total joint replacement. You have
gathered the information you need
to be comfortable that you have made the correct decisions
about the surgery, your surgeon, and the hospital. You have
undergone the appropriate pre-admission preparation. And
you have organized your life and your family, social, and business obligations to optimize your recovery. It is time to focus
on the events of the day of surgery.

That day will begin with your arrival at the hospital,
usually very early in the morning. The check-in process, which
makes sure your pre-operative preparation is complete and
accurate, may take an hour. Your family can usually stay with
you during these first moments of your hospitalization.

Once you have been registered and donned a surgical
gown, you will be wheeled on a cart to the pre-operative holding area. You usually have to say good-bye to your family at
this point, for the hospital and surgical staff needs to do a
number of tasks relatively quickly to prepare you for surgery.

An
Overview
of the
Surgical
Procedure

In the pre-operative holding area, one or more intravenous catheters are placed into veins in your arms. The anesthesiologist updates him- or herself on your health status and reviews your laboratory tests and anesthetic needs. You may be asked to sign the surgical and anesthesiology consent forms at this time. You may then be given medication to help you become more relaxed. When you and your surgical, anesthesia, nursing, and operating room teams are ready, you will be wheeled into the operating room.

The bustle around you will increase once you are placed on the operating room table. The anesthesiologist begins administering your anesthetic. The surgical staff positions instrument trays, which have been opened and checked prior to your arrival, and prepares the urinary catheter that will be inserted after you are anesthetized. The surgical staff also attaches devices to the operating table that will position you and your leg after the anesthetic takes effect. The members of the surgical team put on surgical scrubs for the total joint procedure and wash their hands.

The procedure itself, described in the next pages, usually takes one to three hours. Once completed, the surgical wound will be covered with a dressing, a splint may be applied to your leg, the anesthesia will be discontinued, and you will be carefully transferred to the bed that you will use during your hospital stay. You will then be taken to the recovery room where you are likely to remain for an hour or two. During that time, the anesthetic will start to wear off and you will begin to receive pain medication. Finally, you will be moved to your room and to the care of your inpatient hospital staff.

You will tolerate the day's experience much more easily if you generally understand what it will feel like and what will actually be happening during your procedure. In this chapter, we provide you with a look at the typical surgical day and with Ron's experience with surgery.

Most patients undergoing total joint replacement surgery are admitted to the hospital on the morning of surgery. You need to find out ahead of time from your surgeon which of your medications, if any, you should take on the morning of surgery. Insist that any discrepancies between the anesthesiologist's and surgeon's instructions about these medications be resolved well before your day of surgery.

The pre-operative preparation for a total joint replacement is, in general, no different from that for any procedure requiring a general or regional anesthetic. There are, however, a few aspects of the preparation before surgery that are particularly important for patients undergoing total joint replacement surgery.

As we discussed in Chapter 5, if you have recently developed any symptoms of infection, such as a toothache, or noticed any changes in the appearance of your leg to be operated on, you must call this to the attention of the staff in the pre-operative waiting area. Because infection is the most serious potential complication following a total joint replacement, any signs of a potential source of infection must be evaluated pre-operatively, even as late as the morning of surgery.

You or a relative will probably have given blood should you need a transfusion. Remind the staff in the pre-operative preparation area that such blood is available. The staff will then locate this blood to be sure it is ready and available if you should need it.

Although all hospitals take precautions to correctly identify the joint to be operated upon, it never hurts to remind the staff which leg and which joint is having the surgery. Finally, be sure to give the surgeon instructions about whom he or she should talk to after the operation. Friends and family are concerned not only that the surgery has been performed successfully and safely, but also that you will be correctly cared for in the hospital and at home. Once family and friends learn from the surgeon that you have gone through your surgery, they can begin to focus more effectively on what your needs will be following surgery and how they can help meet those needs.

The Morning of Surgery

A Patient's Perspective: Ron

Facing major surgery, especially for the first time, can be quite traumatic. You must deal psychologically with the known risks, such as the risk of harm from anesthesia, but more difficult still is dealing with what you don't know: How painful will this be? Will I be able to handle it? And so on. The combined effect of these concerns can be like an anchor, weighing you down. Don't be surprised if, as you move toward the surgical date, you start to feel a little depressed and unable to cope readily with life's daily challenges. You may also find it difficult to concentrate on your daily tasks or to sleep. I had these reactions, and they are perfectly natural reactions to a highly traumatizing experience.

You can do many things to reduce your stress during the preoperative time. An easy one, which is tremendously helpful, is simply to be aware of what is going on. You can also try to reorganize your life in various ways. If possible, for example, you might try to organize your professional responsibilities so that no critical events are scheduled during the two weeks or so prior to surgery. If you develop sleep disturbance problems, various kinds of assistance are available. Consult your family doctor and go from there.

You probably will be particularly anxious the night before surgery. In almost all cases, you will be spending that night at home and will have to get up at an ungodly hour in the morning to be at the hospital to prepare for surgery. It is particularly important to get a good night's sleep before surgery so you are well rested. I asked my internist to prescribe a mild sedative, which he did. He also suggested that I take one immediately upon waking before going to the hospital. This was very good advice, in my opinion, because the hours immediately preceding surgery can be very difficult. You will be in a room, perhaps with a family member, waiting for an orderly to come and get you for surgery. You will be quite nervous. Out of an excess of caution, virtually no hospital will provide you with even a mild sedative to calm your nerves at this early point. Your family doctor might, but if you do take one, *be sure to tell the hospital staff exactly what and how much you've taken.*

Once the orderly comes for you, you will be taken to the surgical holding area where various preparations occur. It will be a relief to you to have things underway. The staff that you meet in this area will be quite experienced and will be sensitive to both your physical and psychological needs. At some point you will be asked if you'd like a sedative. If you took something before coming to the hospital, convey that information, and then tell them you would like whatever they can provide. There is no point to suffering in silence at this stage. I recommend that you get as comfortable as you can, as soon as you can.

Anesthesia for Total Joint Surgery

Patients undergoing total joint surgery frequently fear the prospect of going under anesthesia more than the potential pain of the surgical procedure. The entire health care team must recognize this and deal directly with this concern. Patients should be fully informed about the nature of the anesthetic experience they are going to have. Essentially three types of anesthesia may be used during joint replacement surgery: general, regional, and combined.

General Anesthesia

When a general anesthetic is given, the patient is asleep during the surgery. Both intravenous and inhaled anesthetics are used to relax the brain, muscles, and nerves so the patient feels no pain and has no movement or conscious memory of the surgical procedure.

Regional Anesthesia

Regional anesthesia, or regional block, anesthetizes the nerves leading to the leg being operated upon, thereby eliminating the patient's ability to feel pain during the procedure. Patients occasionally confuse *regional* anesthesia with *local* anesthesia. In the former, the entire leg or region is anesthetized. In the latter, only the nerves in the immediate, local area are anesthetized.

Of the many types of regional anesthesia, some, such as spinal anesthesia, eliminate both the ability to feel and move the leg. Others, such as epidural anesthesia, eliminate only the ability to feel the leg. Epidural anesthesia is the type of regional anesthesia most commonly used in total joint surgery. Regional anesthesia can be used for both total hip and total knee replacement surgery. However, it is probably more frequently used in total knee surgery.

An attractive aspect of regional anesthesia is that it can be used to provide relief of the pain after surgery. For example, epidural anesthesia is usually administered through a catheter placed into the epidural space surrounding the spinal cord. The catheter is left in place during the surgical procedure, and then a dose of long-acting analgesic (pain medication) can be given at the conclusion of the total joint replacement procedure, just before the catheter is removed. This procedure can provide excellent pain relief for twelve to twenty-four hours after the surgery. Alternatively, the epidural catheter can be left in place for the day or two following surgery and analgesics can be administered through it.

Combined Anesthesia

THE THIRD TYPE OF ANESTHESIA used in total joint replacement surgery combines aspects of both general and regional anesthesia. In this type of anesthesia, an epidural catheter is placed prior to starting the total joint procedure, and the anesthetic is administered in the usual way. A light general anesthetic is then given. The advantages of this combined approach are threefold. *First,* the effects of the general anesthetic make the patient oblivious to the procedure. This may be particularly helpful in total hip surgery, where patients usually lie on their sides for a number of hours. It may also be attractive to patients who are concerned about hearing the conversations and noises in the operating room. *Second,* substantially less general anesthetic agent is needed in the combined approach, and thus there is less risk involved. This may be very helpful in patients who have medical conditions, such as severe lung disease, which might make a general anesthetic more risky. *Third,* the combined approach also facilitates the administration of analgesia following surgery, as described previously.

Patients frequently ask their surgeon which anesthetic he or she prefers. Surgeons rarely have a preference. If they do, they will probably make this preference known directly to the anesthesiologist. Patients, however, often have a preference about their anesthesia and should feel comfortable expressing these preferences to their surgeon and anesthesiologist. Make sure to discuss with your surgeon and anesthesiologist the options available to you well before your day of surgery so you don't feel pressured to choose a type of anesthesia immediately before you go into the operating room.

A T SOME POINT BEFORE the day of surgery, you will talk to an anesthesiologist from the hospital who will discuss options with you and put together a plan for you. However, not until you are moved to the surgical holding area will you meet the anesthesiologist who is actually handling your case. My experience has been that the anesthesiologist on call the day of your operation may or may not agree with that plan, which frankly I find highly unacceptable. If you have a strong desire for a certain type of anesthesia, and if the hospital is willing to accept that, a single doctor should not disregard your choice. In one of my operations, for example, I planned to use an epidural catheter for post-operative pain relief. The anesthesiologist refused to commit to doing so, even though I had discussed this thoroughly with the hospital's anesthesia department representatives. In the future, I intend to ensure this won't happen again. If all else fails, you can refuse to proceed until the issue is resolved to your satisfaction.

One last word about anesthesia. I tried a regional block for one of the operations and quickly decided it would not work. The description of your position during the operation does not convey how uncomfortable it is if you are awake during the surgery. You are not only on your side for up to five hours; you are also pinned in a holding device that puts enormous pressure on your stomach and back. As we were preparing for my first operation, I was put in this position and immediately realized that it would be intolerable to me for an extensive period of time. You may be more tolerant of such matters than I am, but go into this with your eyes open. If you want to try a regional, go ahead, but if it turns out to be too uncomfortable, accept a general or combined.

A Patient's Perspective: Ron

The Goal of Joint Replacement Surgery

THE PRINCIPAL GOAL OF THE joint replacement surgery itself is to replace the rough surfaces of the arthritic joint with smooth, durable implants. Many patients envision total joint surgery as an amputation of their arthritic joint. This frightening concept often discourages patients from seeking this surgical treatment, even though it may be appropriate. The joint resurfacing, although slightly different for hip replacements than for knee replacements, retains all the important structural parts of a patient's limb, including the bones, muscles, tendons, and ligaments. Your limb, including the affected joint, will look normal after a total joint replacement. (See Figures 6-1 and 6-2.)

right,
FIGURE 6-1
Hip Replacement

A twenty-year-old hip replacement with no evidence of failure (loosening or wear).

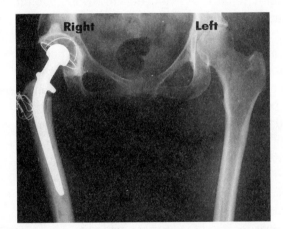

below,
FIGURE 6-2
Knee Replacement

A. *A sixty-year-old woman with osteoarthritis of her left knee, prior to knee replacement surgery.*

B. *Same patient ten years after the knee replacement, with no evidence of failure (loosening or wear).*

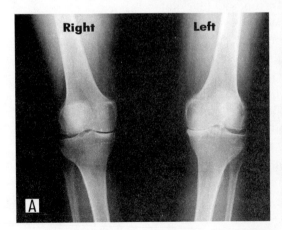

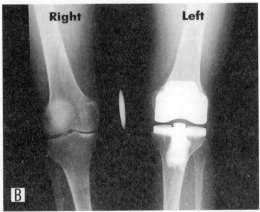

The term *total* joint replacement means that *all* of the rough surfaces of the arthritic joint are covered or replaced by the implant. Thus, the femoral head is replaced and the acetabulum is resurfaced in a *total hip* replacement. The end of the femur, the top of the tibia, and the undersurface of the patella are resurfaced in a *total knee* replacement.

Many parts of the total hip and total knee replacement surgical procedures are similar, including the types of anesthesia that are used, the preparation of the patient in the pre-operative waiting room, the tools that are used to prepare the bones for the implants, and the care of the patient in the recovery room. However, the two procedures do have important differences in the ways that the implants are positioned and attached to the bones.

The Total Hip Replacement Procedure

ONCE THE ANESTHETIC HAS BEEN successfully administered and a catheter has been inserted into the urinary bladder, patients undergoing total hip replacements are usually placed on their sides for the procedure. As Ron described, they are held on their sides by special positioners. A primary, or first time, total hip replacement usually takes one to three hours. Spending this much time on your side, firmly held by hip positioners, might leave you a bit sore for a few days on the side you lie on during your surgery or in your lower back. While Ron found this position extremely uncomfortable, many patients (about half of those who have the procedure), use a regional anesthetic and tolerate being positioned on their sides without particular difficulty.

Making the Incision

A TYPICAL INCISION OF SIX to twelve inches is made along the outer side of the upper part of your leg and buttock being operated on. The actual length and location of the incision may depend on many factors unique to your case, including the type of procedure being performed, the type of prosthesis being used, your size, and the type of arthritis and the associated deformity present. Many different surgical approaches to the

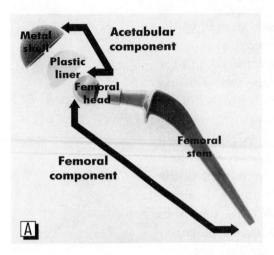

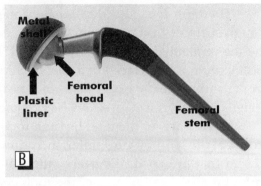

FIGURE 6-3

Prosthetic Components for the Hip

A. *An unassembled modular total hip implant.*

B. *An assembled modular total hip implant.*

hip joint can be carried out through several given incisions. Thus, you will not be able to tell from your incision exactly which surgical approach was used to insert your total hip.

The actual surgical approach used by your surgeon will be the one he or she is most familiar with and can perform most effectively and safely. The approach is not implant specific. Identical implants can be successfully inserted through different surgical approaches. In most primary total hip replacements, the surgical approach cuts very little muscle. Thus, in general, total hip replacements are not particularly painful procedures and are not particularly debilitating. Muscle rehabilitation can be initiated very soon after surgery.

Inserting the Prosthetic Components

THE ACETABULAR, OR CUP, COMPONENT of a total hip replacement is usually inserted first. (See Figure 6-3.) Because the acetabular component is usually hemispherical or elliptical, the surgeon must reshape your acetabulum, which is usually not quite hemispherical. He or she does this using instruments called reamers which are attached to an air-, gas-, or battery-powered device that looks like a drill. The reamers come in many different sizes. The surgeon uses progressively larger reamers until he or she reaches the size that fits your acetabulum exactly. A trial implant is then positioned in the prepared acetabulum to be sure that the fit is correct and the cup is appropriately oriented.

As with all total joint implants, the goal of acetabular preparation is to ensure that the component is (1) securely fixed to the bone, (2) properly aligned with the bone, and (3) placed so that the soft tissue tension is correct. Longevity and function of this component, like all total joint implants, depends on these three goals being met. Surgeons often use special alignment guides to check both the proposed and final position of the acetabular component. Once the size of the implant has been selected and the desired orientation determined, the actual implant is inserted.

ACETABULAR COMPONENTS CAN BE INSERTED with or without cement. *Cemented implants* are usually all polyethylene (plastic). *Uncemented implants* consist of a metal-backing and polyethylene insert. The surgeon securely fixes a cemented cup by precisely preparing bone, carefully mixing the cement, correctly applying the cement to bone, and accurately inserting the cup into cement.

An uncemented acetabular component is securely fixed by inserting the metal shell so it fits tightly within the cavity created by the reamers. This tight fit assures that bone will grow onto and into the surface of the implant. The metal backings of uncemented cups have specially prepared surfaces onto which bone can grow. These surfaces are usually either porous or a material that stimulates bone to attach to the metal shell.

Once the acetabular component is inserted, any bone protruding over the edge of the cup is trimmed to prevent the femoral component, which is about to be inserted, from rubbing against these protrusions and being dislocated from the cup.

Femoral components can also be inserted with or without cement. If the femoral component is to be inserted *with cement*, the intramedullary canal, the part of bone that contains bone marrow, is opened and cleared of loose bone fragments,

Securing the Prosthetic Components

marrow, and blood. The size of the implant that is most appropriate can then be determined. In determining the size of the implant, the surgeon must allow for space around the implant for the cement.

Once the surgeon selects the size of the cemented implant, he or she determines the correct leg length and selects the correct femoral head-neck length. Then the surgeon is ready to cement the actual component.

This is the critical step for achieving rigid, durable fixation of a cemented femoral stem. The femoral canal is thoroughly cleaned and dried, so no blood will be present between the cement and bone. To hold the implant securely, the cement must actually penetrate the bone, which it cannot do if blood is covering the surface of the bone.

Once the cement is injected into the femur, the actual implant is inserted into the cement. Bone cement takes ten to fifteen minutes to harden. Once this has occurred, the femoral implant is rigidly fixed in bone and can withstand virtually any amount of weight bearing.

Implant insertion is concluded by the surgeon selecting the femoral head that gives the most stable reduction and provides the best soft tissue tension. Usually, this is the femoral head selected during the trial reduction described earlier.

If the femoral component is to be inserted *without cement*, the surgeon prepares the femur somewhat differently than just described. The goal of the insertion of an uncemented femoral component is to achieve such rigid fixation of the implant within the femur so that (1) it will not move, even with immediate, maximum weight bearing; and (2) bone will grow onto the implant to provide enduring secure fixation. To accomplish this, the surgeon must be sure that part or all of the implant fits exactly within the femur. The surgeon determines the size and shape of the implant that will fill it most precisely. When the femoral component is being inserted without cement, the surgeon must be careful to avoid fracturing the femur as he or she prepares the femur for the very tightly fitting implant. Once the uncemented implant is successfully inserted, the remainder of the femoral preparation is carried out identically to the preparation for the cemented component.

ONCE THE FEMORAL AND ACETABULAR COMPONENTS are inserted, the surgeon closes the wound. To make sure the femoral head will remain secure within the acetabulum after surgery, the surgeon reattaches all soft tissues that were detached during operation. To prevent a wound infection, the surgeon makes sure all the layers of tissue that were opened are accurately and securely closed and that there is no contact between the skin, on which many types of bacteria grow, and the hip joint. A sterile dressing is applied after the closure. This dressing absorbs any bloody drainage that might occur immediately after surgery and prevents the drainage from being contaminated by bacteria on the skin.

Closing the Incision

A S IN TOTAL HIP REPLACEMENT SURGERY, the surgeon performing a total knee replacement must securely fix the implant to the bones, make sure the devices are properly aligned, and restore the soft tissue—that is, ligaments and muscles—to their proper tension. In both total hip and knee replacement surgeries, failure to fix the implants rigidly to the bone and align the implants properly causes pain for the patient and early failure of the prostheses. In total hip surgery, failure to balance the soft tissues properly may lead to a dislocation of the hip. In total knee surgery, however, failure to balance the soft tissues properly may lead to a joint that not only feels unstable but also is unstable.

Three components are usually inserted during the total knee replacement: the femoral, tibial, and patella (kneecap) segments. The order in which the bones are prepared for these implants may vary according to a surgeon's preference. (See Figure 6-4.)

The Total Knee Replacement Procedure

FIGURE 6-4
*Prosthetic Components
for the Knee*

A. *An unassembled
modular total knee
implant.
Left: posterior cruciate
retaining model.
Right: posterior cru-
ciate sacrificing model.*

B. *A modular total
knee implant in
position of function.*

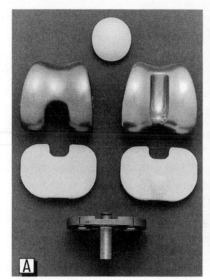
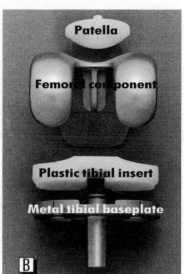

Instruments

THE MOST DRAMATIC ADVANCEMENT in total knee replacement surgery since the 1980s has been the development of
instruments that make it possible for surgeons to implant
prostheses accurately and reproducibly. These instruments
are much more complex than those used for the typical total
hip replacement. As many as ten trays of relatively heavy
pieces of equipment may have to be available for a routine
total knee replacement.

The instruments used for a total knee replacement ensure that the bone cuts are correctly oriented and accurate.
The instruments help the surgeon convert a leg that often is
crooked—for instance, bowlegged—into one that is straight.
The jig instruments help the surgeon make bone cuts that allow the implants to fit snugly against the bone.

The Three-Part Procedure

THE TOTAL KNEE REPLACEMENT PROCEDURE consists of three
parts: the bone cuts, the balancing of soft tissues, and the fixation of the implants to bone.

The bone cuts for the femur, tibia, and patella must be correctly oriented in the forward-backward, side-to-side, and rotational planes. These cuts, which in the 1980s were usually made virtually freehand, can be made very accurately and reproducibly using the multitude of jigs and alignment guides present in total knee instrumentation sets today. Accurately making these cuts ensures that the leg will be straight at the end of the procedure.

The Bone Cuts

The surgeon balances the soft tissues once he or she makes the bone cuts. Trial implants are placed on the cut bones and the knee is tested to be sure that it can lie completely flat and that it does not have excessive or asymmetric side-to-side or front-to-back motion. The knee is also bent with the trial implants in place to be sure that adequate motion can be obtained and to confirm that the patella will not dislocate. Soft tissue balancing is the most difficult part of the surgical procedure. Currently, instruments equivalent to those used for the bone cuts do not exist to help guide the surgeon in correctly balancing the soft tissues. Accurate soft tissue balancing depends upon the experience and judgment of the surgeon.

Balancing the Soft Tissues

The final step of the total knee replacement procedure, securing the implants to bone, is equivalent to the total hip replacement procedure. However, unlike hip replacements, when virtually all acetabular components and many (perhaps half) femoral components are fixed to bone *without* cement, virtually all total knee components—femur, tibia, and patella—are fixed to bone *with* cement. The character of the femur, tibia, and patella, and the shapes of these bones after cuts have been made favor the use of cement.

Securing the Implants

ONCE THE TOTAL HIP or total knee replacement procedures are complete, you will be transferred to the recovery room and, shortly thereafter, to your room. The procedures are designed to provide you with an implant that will give you pain-free, virtually full function for a very long time.

Conclusion

In a very short time you should be able to start using the therapy techniques that you have been practicing.

The implants and techniques are designed to allow you to start toward this goal almost immediately after recovering from anesthesia. If the surgeon has done his or her job correctly, in a very short time you should be able to start using the therapy techniques that you have been practicing.

 # POST-SURGERY

T HE POST-OPERATIVE PERIOD is crucial to the success of hip and knee surgery. Your surgeon, your physical therapist, the hospital staff, and you have things to attend to, ranging from controlling pain and infection, to beginning rehabilitation, to making preparations for going home. We encourage you to be actively involved in all these matters, but frankly it is not easy to muster the energy and concentration that you need to deal with everything in those first few days following surgery.

Some of the factors that will lessen your normal capacity for purposeful action and planning are simply unavoidable, such as the restrictions on mobility and the necessity of pain medication (which can reduce your ability to concentrate). The solution to this problem is knowledge. The more you understand what is going on, the quicker and more efficient your recovery will be. This chapter explains what the post-operative period is like, what will be done and why, and the implications of different aspects of your care.

Recovering from Total Hip and Knee Replacement Surgery

AFTER YOU HAVE SPENT an hour or two in the recovery room, you will be moved back to your hospital room. If your physicians determine that it is safest to keep you in a monitored bed following surgery, you may spend a day in the intensive care unit (ICU) before going to your hospital room.

Most people are surprised by the speed at which they are expected to recover after their surgery. You may believe that your physicians, nurses, and therapists are cruel for pushing you to get up, walk, and eat when you feel barely conscious. For the first few days after surgery, you may feel as if you have been hit by a train. The intravenous catheters, bladder catheter, blood draws, injections, splints, dressings, and variety of medical interventions may overwhelm you. However, the faster you are up and around, the faster you will recover.

Care Protocols

MOST HOSPITALS HAVE STANDARD PROTOCOLS of care for patients who have undergone joint replacement surgery. These care protocols, or clinical pathways, list all the medical and rehabilitation interventions and patient goals for each day of the hospital stay, starting from the moment you are wheeled out of the operating room. Examples of the care protocol given to patients at our medical center are shown in Figures 7-1 and 7-2.

FIGURE 7-1: Hip Replacement Care Protocol
Day 1 • Date _____

What To Expect:

❏ You will return from surgery to your bed.

❏ You may receive blood transfusions (your own) after surgery and within the next two days.

❏ You may have reinfusion of the blood from your surgical drain.

❏ You will have daily blood tests.

❏ A compression device on your feet or legs to improve circulation and prevent blood clots.

❏ A catheter (tube) to drain your urine for about 2 days.

❏ IV's, antibiotics, and a blood thinner.

❏ Medication for pain relief. This may be given by epidural, PCA (IV), injection, pills.

What To Do:

❏ Use your spirometer and cough 10 times every hour everyday.

❏ Use your PCA as frequently as you need to for pain relief.

❏ Let the nurse know how your pain medication is working. Rate your pain on a scale of 0—10 with 0 meaning no pain and 10 the worst pain you could imagine:

No Pain				Moderate Pain				Worst Pain		
0	1	2	3	4	5	6	7	8	9	10

❏ Take sips of water/ice chips and clear liquids. Eat regular food gradually starting tomorrow.

❏ Call the nurse to help you change position from your back to your unoperated side once in a while.

❏ Keep the abduction splint between your legs.

❏ Wear your compression boots at all times.

Hip Replacement Care Protocol : Day 2 • Date _____

What To Expect:

❑ Your nurse and PT will assist you to sit at the edge of your bed, stand with a walker, take a few steps, and sit in a chair.

❑ Physical therapy every day.

❑ Your drain may be discontinued.

❑ A visit from the social worker or discharge planner to discuss your discharge plans.

What To Do:

❑ Use your spirometer and cough 10 times every hour everyday.

❑ Use your PCA as needed for pain relief. Tell your nurse how you would rate your pain throughout the day.

❑ Keep the abduction splint between your legs.

❑ Remember your hip precautions!
  • Don't turn your foot/leg in.
  • Don't twist your body.
  • Don't cross your legs.
  • Don't bend over so you're more than 90 degrees flexion at the hips.

❑ Take the medication tonight that will help prevent you from getting constipated.

Hip Replacement Care Protocol : Day 3 • Date _____

What To Expect:

❏ Your wound drain and urine catheter will be removed. We will encourage you to walk to the bathroom. You will have to use a raised toilet seat.

❏ Your PCA and IV's will be removed. You will receive pills for pain relief.

❏ To sit up in a chair twice today. You may start walking with a walker/crutches.

❏ A visit from the occupational therapist (OT).

❏ If you are going to a rehab facility you may be able to go today or tomorrow.

What To Do:

❏ Talk with your doctor/nurse about discharge plans (home or rehab).

❏ Let your nurse know how the pain medicine is working. Ask for pain medication before pain is at "10."

❏ Drink a lot of fluids so you can urinate. Begin to eat regular diet.

❏ Start walking to the bathroom with help—no more bedpans! Don't forget to use the raised toilet seat.

❏ Remember your hip precautions!
  • Don't turn your foot/leg in.
  • Don't twist your body.
  • Don't cross your legs.
  • Don't bend over so you're more than 90 degrees flexion at the hips.

Hip Replacement Care Protocol : Day 4 • Date _____

The worst is over; it's all downhill from here! We will help you to accomplish these goals so you will be ready to go home as soon as possible.

What to Expect:

❑ A test to rule out blood clots in your legs.

❑ The OT will teach you how to bathe and dress the lower half of your body using your hip precautions. Before you go home, you will be taught how to get in and out of a bathtub and car safely.

❑ Your nurse will begin to review your discharge instructions with you.

❑ If you haven't already had a bowel movement you will receive some medication to help with this.

❑ You may start going to the gym for further therapy and exercises. Your physical therapy goals are:
   • Walking safely with crutches.
   • Going up and down stairs or stepping on and off a curb safely.
   • Increasing the strength in your leg and hip muscles.

❑ Your therapists will review your home exercise and safety program with you before you go home.

❑ Before you go home you should be able to:
   • Demonstrate your home exercise program.
   • Tell us what your activity restrictions (including hip precautions) and goals are.
   • Tell us how you will take care of your incision and new hip.
   • Tell us how you would identify an infection or blood clot and when you would call the doctor.
   • Tell us about your anticoagulation therapy (blood thinner).

❑ Before you go home, arrangements will be made for removal of your staples.

What To Do:

❑ Take your pain medication regularly so you can participate in therapy with the least amount of pain. Let your nurse know how well your pain is being managed.

❑ Work with PT to reach your goals.

❑ Walk to the bathroom. Walk in the hall with help as often as you can during the day and evening. Sit up for meals.

Day 4 , continued

❏ Start thinking about going home. Discuss your discharge needs with your doctor, nurse, physical therapist, and discharge planner.

❏ Order a raised toilet seat to take home with you.

❏ Use the OT tools to bathe and dress yourself.

❏ Remember your hip precautions.
  • Don't turn your foot/leg in.
  • Don't twist your body.
  • Don't cross your legs.
  • Don't bend over so you're more than 90 degrees flexion at the hips.

❏ You should be able to tell us:
  • What your home exercise program is.
  • What your activity restrictions and expectations are.
  • How to take care of your incision and your new knee.
  • How you would identify an infection or blood clot when you would call the doctor.
  • About your blood thinners.

❏ You may have your staples taken out before you go home. If not, arrangements will be made to have the staples removed later on.

❏ Your OT will show you how to get in and out of a bathtub and car and review some home safety tips with you.

❏ Your PT will review your home program of exercises, transfers, and gait.

Congratulations! You made it this far—Good luck and keep up the good hard work!

FIGURE 7-2: Knee Replacement Care Protocol
Day 1 • Date _____

What To Expect:

❏ You will return from surgery to your bed.

❏ You may have a splint on your operated leg.

❏ You may receive blood transfusions (your own) after surgery and within the next two days as needed.

❏ You may have reinfusion of the blood from your surgical drain.

❏ You will have daily blood tests.

❏ A catheter (tube) to drain your urine for about 2 days.

❏ A compression device on your feet or legs to improve circulation and prevent blood clots.

❏ IV's, medicine for pain relief, antibiotics, and a blood thinner.

❏ You may start using your CPM if your doctor orders it.

❏ Medication for pain relief. This may be given by epidural, PCA (IV), injection, pills.

What To Do:

❏ Use your spirometer and cough 10 times every hour.

❏ If you have a PCA machine, use it as often as needed for pain relief. Let the nurse know how well your pain medication is working. Rate your pain on a scale of 0—10 with 0 meaning no pain and 10 the worst pain you could imagine:

No Pain   *Moderate Pain*   *Worst Pain*

0	1	2	3	4	5	6	7	8	9	10

❏ Take sips of water/ice chips and clear liquids. Hold off on regular food to prevent or decrease nausea.

❏ Call the nurse to help you change position from your back to your unoperated side once in a while.

❏ Wear your compression boots at all times.

Knee Replacement Care Protocol: Day 2 • Date _____

What To Expect:

❑ Your nurse and physical therapist (PT) will help you sit at the edge of the bed and stand with a walker, take a few steps and sit in a chair for a short time.

❑ PT exercises every day.

❑ Your drain (if you had one) may be removed.

❑ A visit from the social worker or discharge planner to discuss your discharge plans.

What To Do:

❑ Use your spirometer and cough 10 times every hour.

❑ Use your PCA as needed for pain relief. Tell your nurse how your pain medicine is working.

❑ Drink plenty of fluids. Try not to take solid/heavy food for 1 full day after surgery

❑ Take the medication offered to you tonight that will help prevent constipation.

Knee Replacement Care Protocol: Day 3 • Date _____

What To Expect:

❑ A visit from the occupational therapist (OT).

❑ Your wound drain and urine catheter will be removed, if not already done. We will encourage you to walk to the bathroom. You may need to use a raised toilet seat (we will provide).

❑ Your PCA or epidural and IV's will be removed. You will receive pills for pain relief.

❑ To sit up in a chair twice today. You will start walking with a walker/crutches, if you haven't already started.

❑ To start using the CPM machine if you haven't already started.

❑ If you are scheduled to go to a rehab facility, you may be able to go tomorrow.

What To Do:

❑ Talk with your doctor/nurse about discharge plans (home or rehab).

❑ Take pain medicine at regular times before your pain is a "10." Let your nurse know how the pain medicine is working.

❑ Drink a lot of fluids so you can urinate. Begin to eat regular diet.

❑ Start walking to the bathroom with help—no more bedpans! Don't forget to use the raised toilet seat.

❑ Continue to take the medication to prevent constipation.

Knee Replacement Care Protocol: Day 4 • Date _____

The worst is over; it's all downhill from here! We will help you to accomplish these goals so you will be ready to go home as soon as possible. You may go home as soon as tomorrow.

What to Expect:

❑ A test to rule out blood clots in your legs.

❑ The OT will teach you how to bathe and dress the lower half of your body. Before you go home, you will be taught how to get in and out of a bathtub and car safely.

❑ Your nurse will begin to review your discharge instructions with you.

❑ If you haven't already had a bowel movement you will receive some medication to help with this.

❑ You may start going to the gym for further therapy and exercises. Your physical therapy goals are:
  • Walking safely with crutches.
  • Going up and down stairs or stepping on and off a curb safely.
  • Increasing the strength in your leg and bending your knee.

❑ Your therapists will review your home exercise and safety program with you before you go home.

❑ Before you go home you should be able to:
  • Demonstrate your home exercise program.
  • Tell us what your activity restrictions and goals are.
  • Tell us how you will take care of your incision and new knee.
  • Tell us how you would identify an infection or blood clot and
    when you would call the doctor. Tell us strategies for preventing a blood clot.
  • Tell us about your anticoagulation therapy (blood thinner).

❑ Before you go home, arrangements will be made for removal of your staples.

What to Do:

❑ Take your pain medication regularly so you can participate in therapy with the least amount of pain. Let your nurse know how well your pain is being managed.

❑ Work with the physical therapist to accomplish your goals.

❑ Use your CPM as much as your doctor, nurse, or physical therapist suggests.

❑ Walk to the bathroom, walk in the hall with assistance as often as you can during the day and evening, sit up for meals.

Day 4 , continued

❏ Start thinking about going home, discuss your discharge needs with your doctor, nurse, physical therapist, and discharge planner.

❏ Order a raised toilet set to take home with you, if needed.

❏ Use the tools from the OT to bathe and dress yourself.

❏ You should be able to tell us:
   • What your home exercise program is.
   • What your activity restrictions and expectations are.
   • How to take care of your incision and your new knee.
   • How you would identify an infection or blood clot when you would call the doctor.
   • About your blood thinners.

❏ You may have your staples taken out before you go home. If not, arrangements will be made to have the staples removed later on.

❏ Your OT will show you how to get in and out of a bathtub and car and review some home safety tips with you.

❏ Your PT will review your home program of exercises, transfers, and gait.

Congratulations! You made it this far—Good luck and keep up the good hard work!

From "Total Knee Replacement: Patient's Path to Recovery," pages 3–8. Reproduced by permission of the Rehabilitation Institute of Chicago and the Northwestern Memorial Hospital, Chicago, Illinois. Copyright © 1994 by Northwestern Memorial Hospital.

ADEQUATE PAIN CONTROL IS A CRITICAL PART of your care. The surgery and rehabilitation are painful, and you will not be able to make good progress in therapy unless the pain is well controlled. For the first forty-eight hours you may receive pain medication through an epidural catheter, through intravenous self-administered analgesic pumps (called patient-controlled analgesia or PCA), or by injections of morphine or related compounds on an as-needed basis. After the first two days, you take most of your pain medication orally. Initially these oral analgesics are likely to contain narcotics like hydrocodone or acetaminophen with codeine, which you can take every three to four hours as needed. You will tolerate therapy and will sleep better if you make sure to *take your pain medication about one hour before therapy and at bedtime*.

It is important to have your pain management program established before you leave the hospital. Do not worry about overusing pain medicine or becoming addicted. Physical addiction to pain medicine in this situation is extremely rare. The alternative situation is more likely the case—patients underuse pain medicine in the hospital and at home and suffer unnecessarily. Your ability to function in the first few weeks after leaving the hospital will depend on strong, effective pain management.

Management of Pain

YOU WILL WAKE UP WITH A CATHETER in your bladder and at least one, maybe more, IVs. Don't worry about the catheter. While it is in, you cannot feel it, and it is a great comfort not to have to worry about urinating the first couple of days following surgery. In my experience, its removal ranged from a slight stinging to being completely pain free, so I would put this worry out of your mind.

The IVs are a different matter. If everything is operating properly, the IVs themselves are painless after insertion, and insertion is not much different from getting a shot. Removal is also completely painless. However, things can go wrong with IVs. I had an IV that caused my forearm to bruise horribly and swell up to twice

A Patient's Perspective: Ron

Catheters and IVs

its normal size. It should have been removed much earlier than it was. The nurses or doctors should have observed what was occurring and taken action, and I should have, too. None of us did, though, and the result was not pretty to behold. It also caused problems. The arm was so swollen that blood could not be taken from it, nor could it be taken from the other arm, either, because that arm still had an IV in it.

Another problem I had was that after a couple of days, the site of the IV was becoming increasingly uncomfortable. I thought this was natural; it wasn't. IVs should not hurt. If yours does, you may need to have it removed and another one started somewhere else. If you feel discomfort at the IV site, bring it to the staff's attention, and insist that action be taken.

Pain Management

In each of my surgeries I woke up in the operating room, but I have two different stories to tell. In the first case, I woke up and was soon in throbbing pain. I got some pain medications from the nurses in the recovery room, but not a lot. I was eventually transferred to my room, where the pain continued. I was falling in and out of consciousness, so I was not in agonizing pain the entire time. But whenever I was awake it hurt badly. I was on a PCA, but the pain control was inadequate. I remember my wife asking for assistance for me and being told, "We can control but not eliminate pain." This experience was consistent with reports published a few years ago that implied that hospitals routinely undermedicated for pain.

Make sure a family member is assertive enough to make the hospital respond if you are obviously seriously uncomfortable.

My most recent operation, the revision on my left hip, was completely different. I again woke up in the operating room, but this time largely pain-free. In the recovery room, when I began to sense pain, I would ask for assistance and I received it each time. The pain was virtually controlled entirely. When I got to my room, I was placed on a PCA, and it worked so well that I was comfortable and slept through most of the night. By the next day, the pain was completely controlled. It still hurt some, and the pain would ebb and flow, but I could control it.

What explains these two different experiences? I really do not know. It may be that pain management has gotten better in general. It may be that things were done differently in the second case. I do think that there is an important lesson for you. Notwithstanding David and Vicky's view that this is not a particularly painful operation, my experience is that it can be quite painful if you are not adequately medicated. And perhaps even more importantly, you or your family may have to see to it that you are medicated. Pain management is a variable that can be handled better or worse, and you and your family may have to insist that it is handled properly. Do so when you plan the operation, and after the operation make sure a family member is assertive enough to make the hospital respond if you are obviously seriously uncomfortable.

Sleep

AFTER HIP AND KNEE REPLACEMENT many people have difficulty sleeping, starting in the hospital and continuing at home. The pain, noise, catheters, dressing changes, hospital bed, and a host of other factors make sleeping in the hospital unbelievably difficult. Nearly all patients use strong sleeping pills in the hospital. When you return home, however, sleep does not come much easier. The newly replaced joint becomes stiff and painful fairly quickly when at rest, and you will have difficulty finding a comfortable position.

We encourage our patients to continue to use sleeping medication, whether by prescription or over the counter, for the first few weeks after surgery. Also important are the sleep habits listed in Table 3-4. Some people are able to avoid sleeping medication and still get restful sleep after surgery using those practices alone.

Immediate Physical and Occupational Therapy

PHYSICAL THERAPY BEGINS on the first post-operative day. The therapist will help you dangle your leg at the side of the bed and also help you attempt to stand with a walker or crutches. You may sit in a chair next to your bed for about one hour. In addition, the therapist will help you begin exercising in bed, using exercises such as ankle pumps, heel slides, and isometric muscle contraction.

By the second post-operative day, you should begin to stand and walk in your room. By this time you should be able to sit in the chair an hour twice a day. The physical therapist will help you perform specific stretching and strengthening exercises. Your Foley catheter will be removed, your IV will be taken out, and you will be started on medications, including laxatives, to return your body to its usual functioning.

On the second post-operative day you will meet your occupational therapist, who will instruct you on safe techniques for dressing, bathing, and toileting. He or she will provide you with adaptive equipment to assist in your self-care skills, such as a long-handled reacher, raised toilet seat, and bath bench (recall these items from Chapter 3).

Therapy progresses quite vigorously until you are ready for discharge. By the third or fourth post-operative day, you should be walking independently, smoothly, and comfortably with a walker or crutches. You should be able to transfer to and from your bed and chair, and you should be able to walk to and use the toilet, dress yourself, and give yourself a sponge bath. It is important that you understand what you should *not* do—your precautions—by the time you leave the hospital. (Chapter 8 discusses these precautions at length.)

Finally, you and your family will receive detailed instructions for home care, including a home exercise program. The typical early post-operative exercise program is shown in Figure 7-3. Following your surgeon's and physical therapist's instructions, you should do these exercises every day. When your surgeon approves progressing to the more advanced program, typically six to eight weeks after the operation, proceed to the exercises in Chapter 8.

CPM Machine Therapy (for the Knee)

After knee replacement, many surgeons prescribe the use of a continuous passive motion (CPM) machine. (See Figure 7-4.) This device gently assists the knee that has been operated on to bend and straighten. The nursing and therapy staff set the amount of flexion and speed. You have a control to stop the device. Although philosophies vary among surgeons about the way CPM machines should be used after total joint replacement surgery, all agree that the machines are at most an adjunct to but *do not* act as a substitute for formal physical therapy. Your surgeon and physical therapist will prescribe the CPM procedures that are best for you.

Ankle pump

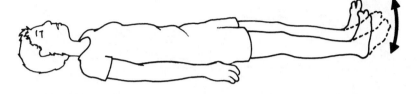

Ankle circle

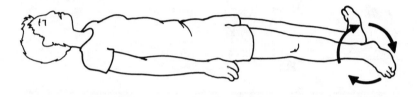

Straight leg raise

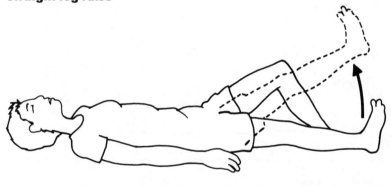

Terminal knee extension

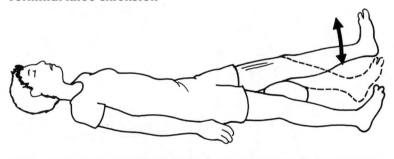

FIGURE 7-3
Early Post-Operative Hip and Knee Replacement Exercise Program

This exercise program for the immediate post-operative period—that is, for the six to eight weeks after surgery—supplements the exercises that you do with your physical therapist. Unless your surgeon or physical therapist instructs you otherwise, perform each exercise on each leg ten to twenty times, twice a day.

CAUTIONS: *Consult your surgeon before performing any of these exercises. Also, if you had a hip replacement, do not lie on your operated side.*

FIGURE 7-3,
continued

Hip extension

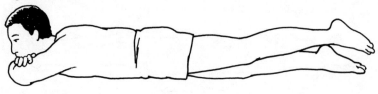

Hip adduction

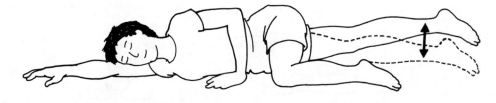

Hip abduction

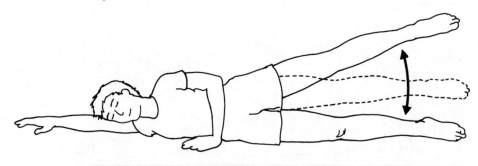

Quadriceps set

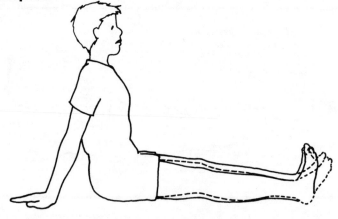

Knee extension

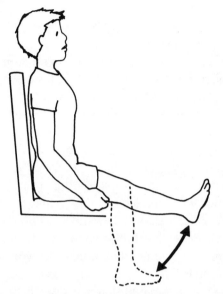

FIGURE 7-3,
continued

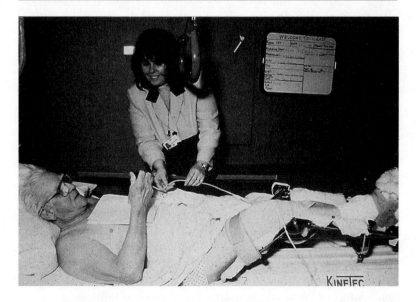

FIGURE 7-4
CPM Machine

The Continuous Passive Motion (CPM) machine slowly bends and straightens a patient's knee following knee surgery.

A Patient's Perspective: Ron

At that moment you cross the bridge from being a person increasingly disabled and caught in a downward spiral to one with a future.

THE MORE ACTIVE YOU ARE THE BETTER, as long as you are sensible about it. It is quite clear to me from my own experience, as well as from watching others in the orthopedic wards, that the sooner you begin to rehabilitate your leg the better. You can begin almost immediately following surgery. As soon as you are able, begin contracting (or tensing) and then relaxing the muscles of your leg. Don't try to move anything, just contract and then relax the muscles and keep doing this as much as you can.

As soon as the hospital staff offers to help you get up to a sitting position with your legs dangling, take them up on the offer. It will feel weird at first, but the weird sensation quickly is replaced with a sense of relief at actually being close to getting out of bed. If the staff feels that you're ready and asks if you want to stand up, try it unless you feel faint. The best thing you can do is to get out of bed, take a step or two, and sit in a chair. The more quickly you do these things—again, as long as you don't feel faint or otherwise ill—the more rapidly you will progress, and the lesser the danger will be from things like clotting.

When you do stand for the first time, it will feel very strange. You will have tubes dangling out of you, although they won't be uncomfortable. You will feel as if a truck ran over you. You will be asked to take a step with a walker or crutches, touching the foot of the leg that was operated on to the ground, but putting no weight on it. You will probably look at the nurse or doctor like he or she is crazy to suggest such an act, but give it a go. The muscles of your leg will actually function. You will be able to move your leg forward and slightly bend your knee. Try it, moving very slowly and carefully, experimenting with your new equipment. It will be strange, but it will work, although within highly defined constraints.

You will be relieved to learn that you can take a step at all, and you will probably notice, as I did, that the pain from your arthritis is completely gone. You may experience, as I did, a great wave of relief. The pain is finally gone. At that moment you cross the bridge from being a person increasingly disabled and caught in a downward spiral from the pain and awkwardness of uncontrollable arthritis to one with a future. You can walk again without pain, admittedly with a walker, but for the first time in who-knows-how-long without pain. Now the only question is how far you can progress. The answer is that you can progress remarkably far.

MOST PATIENTS LEAVE THE HOSPITAL by the fourth or fifth post-operative day, when they are basically independent, caring for themselves but still requiring nursing and therapy interventions, as well as special medications and blood tests. Most hospitals have a social worker, nurse, or discharge planner who will visit you and confirm the arrangements you had made before surgery, revising them as necessary.

Home care arrangements may include a nurse to draw blood, a nurse's aide to help you bathe, and a physical therapist. You will be given specific instructions about your medications, diet, and other important issues such as the possible complications after joint replacement and how to avoid them. Most patients need home or outpatient therapy for at least three to six weeks after surgery to obtain a good functional and physical outcome.

Preparing for Hospital Discharge

DURING YOUR HOSPITAL STAY and for some time afterward, you will receive a number of interventions to prevent the various complications that may occur during the first few days and weeks after hip and knee replacement. Be aware of these potential complications so you can assist in preventing them or alert your physician if signs of them occur.

Complications from Surgery

INFECTION CAN BE A DISASTROUS complication of joint replacement surgery. Fortunately, the incidence of serious infections has been reduced to less than one percent of primary total joint procedures through the use of appropriate pre-operative procedures, specialized operating rooms, strict aseptic technique during surgery, and antibiotics. You will receive antibiotics intravenously to prevent infection for the first twenty-four to forty-eight hours after surgery.

There are two types of infection. Superficial infection is a

Infection

bacterial infection of the tissue just below the skin, while deep infection is a bacterial infection of the joint replacement itself.

Superficial Infections

Superficial infections happen occasionally (approximately five percent of all procedures) and are almost never serious if treated promptly. The main characteristics of superficial wound infections are redness along or near the incision, localized swelling around the incision, and relatively localized pain and tenderness. These signs may be accompanied by small amounts of drainage from the wound. The main danger of superficial wound infections is that, if not promptly and correctly treated, they can extend into the joint replacement and become deep infections. This potential is of particular concern for total knee replacements because the inside of the knee joint is relatively close to the skin.

Wound drainage is not uncommon following a total joint replacement. Most of the time this drainage is sterile and harmless. However, if it persists, a track from the skin to the underlying subcutaneous tissue forms and becomes a conduit whereby skin bacteria can reach and infect this tissue. Sterile, harmless drainage can be easily distinguished from infected drainage by the appearance of the wound and the drainage itself, the smell, and if necessary, a wound culture.

As long as a surgical wound is draining, it should be kept clean and covered with a sterile bandage. You should not expose the wound to the pressure of a shower until all drainage has stopped. You should never hesitate to tell your surgeon about any drainage. Most superficial wound infections can be treated with careful cleansing and dressing of the wound. Your physician may choose to place you on antibiotics. Occasionally, he or she may recommend that the wound be reopened, surgically cleared of infected or dead tissue, and re-sutured. If promptly and effectively treated, superficial wound infections rarely result in deep wound infections and rarely recur.

Deep Infections

Deep wound infections, those involving the joint replacement itself, are extremely serious. The presence of such infections can jeopardize the future of your implant. Fortunately, deep wound infections are exceedingly rare. Deep wound infections can occur very soon after surgery (acute) or months to years after the total joint replacement (late).

Acute deep wound infections occur in less than one percent of primary total joint procedures. Their incidence is slightly higher in revision procedures. The signs of acute deep wound infections, which occur within the first few weeks after surgery, include generalized swelling and redness of the entire joint area (thigh or knee), substantial pain, and possibly a number of systemic signs and symptoms including fever, chills, and malaise. There is frequently, but not always, drainage from the surgery site.

The treatment of an acute deep wound infection will depend upon many factors and requires particularly careful judgment by the surgeon. Because bleeding or excessively zealous exercise, for instance, can cause swelling, redness, and pain near a joint replacement, you need to contact your surgeon if these signs occur.

Deep wound infections can also occur months or years following your surgery. These late infections almost always result from untreated infections from elsewhere in your body spreading to the joint replacement. These can be as, or more, serious than acute deep wound infections. Almost all late infections can be prevented by prompt, correct treatment of the original infection. Therefore, your surgeon will recommend that you take a number of steps to prevent such infections from occurring or spreading.

For example, you should seek immediate treatment for any signs or symptoms of infection, such as urinary frequency or burning. Late infections usually are indicated by pain or instability in a previously well-functioning joint replacement. Both patients and physicians tend to become complacent about the potential for the development of late infection as the years pass following a total joint replacement, particularly if the surgery was successful. It is your responsibility as well as your surgeon's to be vigilant about the potential of this most serious complication.

Prophylactic Antibiotic Treatment

You may be put on antibiotics after joint surgery, just as you may be advised to take antibiotics if you have invasive dental work, a colonoscopy or proctoscopy, or other invasive surgical procedure. Your surgeon should provide you with the details for this prophylactic (preventive) antibiotic treatment.

The significance of having patients take antibiotics prophylactically is a controversial issue in the field. There is no good evidence to support this practice, but there is no good evidence demonstrating that it is ineffective, either. Our judgment is that the risk of infection significantly outweighs the costs and risks of intermittent antibiotic use.

Urinary Retention

A URINARY CATHETER, ALSO CALLED a Foley catheter, is placed into the bladder during surgery and is left in place for twenty-four to thirty-six hours after surgery. Occasionally, some people have difficulty urinating for the first day or two after the catheter comes out. If this happens to you, it may be necessary for the nurse to intermittently catheterize you until your bladder begins working again. Intermittent catheterization can be uncomfortable. If you experience pain during catheter insertion, you can ask the nurses to use a topical anesthetic jelly (lidocaine) to reduce the discomfort. If you have experienced urinary retention, be aware that you are at slightly increased risk of a urinary tract infection. The signs of such an infection (pain with urination, urgency, increased frequency, or blood in the urine) may not occur until you go home.

Constipation

MANY PEOPLE EXPERIENCE CONSTIPATION after surgery as a result of anesthesia, immobility, and pain medication. Drinking fluids and being as mobile as possible quickly after surgery helps prevent constipation. You will receive stool softeners each day. If you do not have a bowel movement by the second or third post-operative day, you may require a suppository. You can reduce the likelihood of this by eating relatively lightly the day or two before surgery and by using a laxative or gentle enema the day before surgery.

Constipation may be a problem for the first *month* after surgery. Inactivity, pain medication, and iron supplements are the primary reasons patients are still bothered by constipation at home. As long as you are taking narcotic pain medication you may require stool softeners on a daily basis to minimize constipation. Drinking fluids (at least 8 glasses a day), supplementing your diet with fiber (such as using Metamucil daily), and walking regularly are the most effective, and natural, methods to eliminate constipation.

Thromboembolic Disease (Blood Clots)

THROMBOEMBOLIC DISEASE, OR BLOOD CLOTS, of the legs may occur after hip and knee replacement surgery. In patients who receive no preventive measures, the incidence may be as high as seventy percent. Fortunately, there are safe and effective measures to prevent blood clots. These preventive measures are mechanical and pharmaceutical.

The primary mechanical method is physical activity soon after surgery. Sitting on the side of the bed and beginning to stand the day after surgery are good ways to prevent blood clots. Most surgeons also prescribe pneumatic compression devices which wrap around the legs and feet, intermittently fill with air, compress the calves, and force blood up the leg, thereby preventing the pooling of blood that leads to the formation of blood clots.

Blood clotting can be prevented also by using blood thinning medication such as warfarin, heparin, low-molecular weight heparin, and aspirin. Some physicians prescribe these medications for up to six weeks after surgery. Warfarin (or Coumadin) is a common medication used. It thins the blood by interfering with the blood clotting system. Its dosage must be carefully regulated through the use of blood tests (a prothrombin time tested at least twice weekly). Warfarin has a narrow therapeutic window, so the dosage of the drug must be altered fairly frequently. Certain medicines, particularly anti-inflammatory agents, and foods such as those high in Vitamin K can affect the level of warfarin in the blood, and should be avoided while on the medication. (See Table 7-1.)

A number of low-molecular weight heparins, such as enoxaparin (Lovenox), are now available and may be as effective as warfarin in preventing blood clots. The patient injects these drugs beneath the skin twice daily for approximately two weeks following surgery. Low-molecular weight heparins, unlike warfarin, have the advantage of not requiring blood tests to monitor their efficacy or safety. However, these drugs are quite expensive and may cost over twenty dollars a day. They may not be covered by your insurance.

Aspirin is used commonly after knee replacement to prevent blood clots, but it is now considered less effective than warfarin or enoxaparin. It may be useful to take one aspirin daily for four to five weeks after you have finished your course of warfarin or low-molecular weight heparin.

TABLE 7-1 • Foods and Drugs to Avoid While Taking Warfarin

Foods	Drugs
❏ Liver (any kind)	❏ Categories of drugs that can interfere with anti-coagulation therapy
❏ Broccoli	• NSAIDs
❏ Brussels sprouts	• Antibiotics
❏ Cauliflower	• Anticonvulsants
❏ Chickpeas	• Antidepressants
❏ Kale	• Oral hypoglycemic medicines
❏ Spinach	• Numerous others
❏ Turnip greens	❏ Vitamins
	❏ Oral contraceptives
	❏ Alcohol

If you are taking warfarin, consult your physician about possible conflicts with any other medications you are taking and about foods you should avoid, such as those listed above.

A Patient's Perspective: Ron

CLOTTING IS A SERIOUS PROBLEM and you need to take it seriously, but the pneumatic compression cuffs are a mixed blessing. I was able to wear them through the first night following surgery, but not thereafter. They are noisy and can be uncomfortable. Try as I might, I could not sleep after the first night with the cuffs, and so I removed them. Some people find them completely comfortable, indeed like them, and are not as distracted by their noise as I was. If you can tolerate them, you should. If they are causing you significant discomfort, as they did me, consult your doctor. If he or she thinks you are particularly susceptible to clots, you should do everything you can to reduce the risk, including losing a little sleep due to the cuffs. If you are not susceptible, have been active during the day, and things are going well, you might be able to forego them.

Dislocation of the Hip

DISLOCATION OF THE KNEE following total joint replacement surgery is a rare, unlikely complication. Dislocation of the hip is far more common.

Because the muscles and soft tissues surrounding the hip joint are weakened by total hip replacement surgery, patients have an increased risk of dislocating a prosthetic hip joint in the first six to eight weeks after the procedure. To prevent this from happening, your surgeon will give you strict precautions against certain motions of the hip that you must follow for six to twelve weeks after surgery.

The specific precautions may depend upon many factors, including the surgical approach, the type of procedure (primary or revision), the pre-existing hip condition, and the rate of your progress with physical therapy. For example, the standard recommendations for the frequently used posterior-lateral surgical approach in a primary total hip replacement are to avoid (1) bending (flexing) the hip more than ninety degrees, (2) crossing (adducting) the legs, and (3) turning the operated leg inward (internal rotation).

The greatest risk for dislocation is during the first two weeks after surgery. Therefore, you may be asked to wear a triangular-shaped brace, called an abductor splint, between your legs while you are in bed at the hospital. When you go home, sleep with a pillow between your legs for the first six to twelve weeks after surgery.

While in the hospital, the occupational therapist and nurses will show you how to dress, bathe, and use the toilet so you can avoid excessive bending at the waist or rotating the leg. Special adaptive equipment, such as a raised toilet seat, reacher, and sock donner, will help you perform your daily routines safely. Avoid sitting in low chairs or soft couches, getting into the tub, and getting into low, small cars with bucket seats for the first two to three months after surgery. (These precautions are summarized in Figure 7-5.)

Nerve Injuries

OCCASIONALLY, INJURY TO A NERVE occurs during surgery, especially during revision procedures or difficult surgeries. If a nerve injury occurs, you will feel pain or numbness along the leg or on the surface of the foot, and weakness of the leg or foot. Most nerve injuries are the result of pressure on the nerve or stretching of the nerve rather than its actually being cut. Consequently, the injuries frequently resolve; however, this healing process may take up to two years.

While most nerve injuries occur during the procedure, some develop in the first few days after surgery. If you notice weakness and numbness in your leg, alert your surgeon immediately. The presence of a nerve injury may delay progress in physical therapy, including walking, and can be very painful. If the injury is associated with weakness in the foot, a special plastic brace may be necessary.

Heterotopic Ossification

HETEROTOPIC OSSIFICATION, also called ectopic bone or myositis ossificans, is abnormal bone deposit in the soft tissue and can occur after hip replacement surgery. Although seen on some x-rays, it rarely causes physical or functional problems. It may cause pain or limited motion at the hip joint.

FIGURE 7-5 • Precautions to Follow for a Total Hip Replacement

All hip replacement patients must follow these three rules until their doctors tell them not to.

Precaution 1: Do not move your operated hip toward your chest (flexion/bending) any more than 90 degrees.

DOs

❏ *Do* sit in a high (17–18 inch seat height), firm arm chair (see *A*, below); use cushions or pillows to make the seat higher if necessary. (*Hint:* To get up from a chair, move to the front edge of the seat, stick out your operated leg, and push yourself to a standing position with your arms. Keep your back straight; don't bend.)

❏ *Do* use a raised toilet seat. Use the toilet marked for handicapped when you go out.

DON'Ts

❏ *Do not* lean forward to get up from a chair or toilet seat. (See *B*, below.)

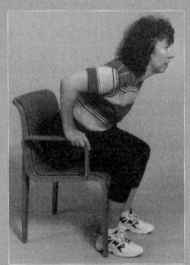

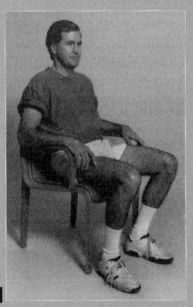

❑ *Do* use your reacher, long-handled shoe horn, and sock aid. (See *C* and *D*, below.)

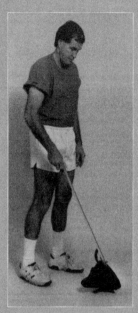

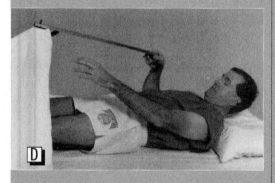

❑ *Do not* bend over to pick up objects, put on your socks and shoes, or pull up your bed covers. (See *E* and *F*, below.)

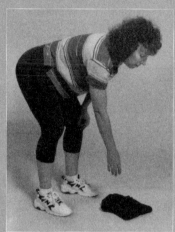

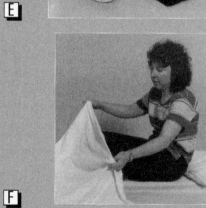

❑ *Do not* raise your legs or knees when sitting or lying down. (See *G*, below.)

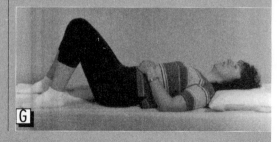

Precaution 2: Do not put your knees and legs together or cross your legs. (See J, K, and M, below and on following page.)

DOs

- ❏ *Do* keep a pillow or the abduction splint between your legs when sitting in a chair or lying in bed. (See *H, I,* and *L,* below and on following page.)

DON'Ts

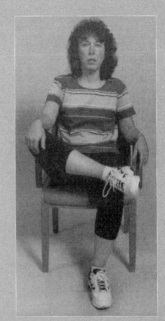

J

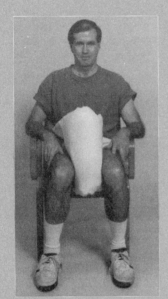

H

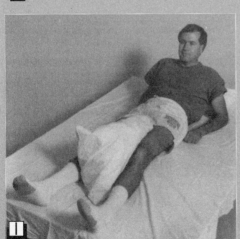

I

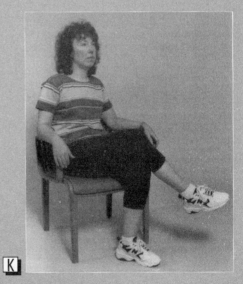

K

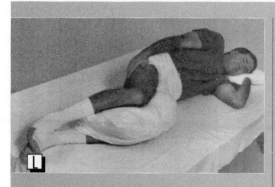

❑ (But *do not* turn onto the healing/
   operated side.)

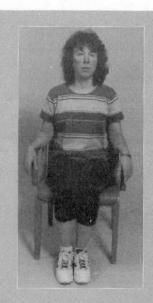

Precaution 3: Do not turn the operated leg's foot or knee inward. (See N, below.)

DO:

❑ *Do* keep everything in easy reach and
   in front of you.

❑ *Do* keep your legs apart and your knee
   and toes on the operated side pointing
   up or straight ahead.

DON'T:

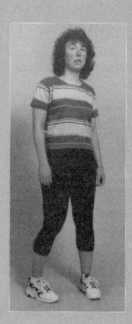

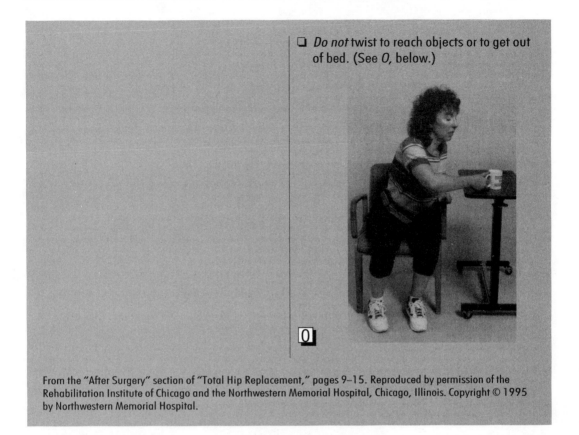

❏ *Do not* twist to reach objects or to get out of bed. (See *O,* below.)

From the "After Surgery" section of "Total Hip Replacement," pages 9–15. Reproduced by permission of the Rehabilitation Institute of Chicago and the Northwestern Memorial Hospital, Chicago, Illinois. Copyright © 1995 by Northwestern Memorial Hospital.

Certain people, such as those with the medical condition ankylosing spondylitis or DISH syndrome, may be at higher risk to develop heterotopic ossification. Such patients may be treated with anti-inflammatory medications or low-dose irradiation.

Leg Length Discrepancies (in the Hips)

AN ISSUE IMPORTANT to patients is whether or not their legs will be the same length after hip replacement. Many patients with an arthritic hip feel that their affected leg is shorter than their unaffected leg. They look forward to having legs that will be the same length and function better. Some patients may have altered the length of their pant legs or added a lift to their shoe to deal with the discrepancy in leg length, whether real or perceived.

This issue of leg length is substantially more complex than it seems. Most people, with or without arthritis, unknowingly have one leg that is up to one-half of an inch longer than the other.

A hip affected by arthritis may cause the leg to be shorter than the unaffected leg or one that feels shorter. A leg that *feels* like a different length than the other leg but actually is *not* is described as having an *apparent* leg length discrepancy. This apparent discrepancy occurs because the arthritic hip process, including the pain associated with it, causes the leg to be held in a position that is flexed forward, which makes the affected extremity appear to be shorter or longer.

Although the difference between true and apparent leg length discrepancy may not seem important to a patient with a bad hip, it is crucial to the orthopedic surgeon, who is responsible for making the legs as close to equal as possible. If the leg is *truly* different in length because of the hip disease, the hip replacement must make up for the loss in length. If the leg is only *apparently* different in length, then the hip replacement used must only reproduce the current length of the bone.

One of the most important things an orthopedic surgeon will do in planning for your hip surgery is to determine how he or she will deal with your leg length differences, real or apparent. The surgeon must have implants available that will allow correction of the leg length disparity. During the operation, determining the correct leg length involves more than simply measuring the length of the leg and altering the length according to the pre-operative measurements. As discussed in Chapter 6, the surgeon must re-establish the length of the bones during the operation and restore the correct tension of the tissues around the hip. If the soft tissue tension is not restored correctly, the hip replacement may dislocate or feel unstable after surgery. The length of implant necessary to establish correct soft tissue tension may be different (shorter or longer) than the length of the device required to simply restore the length of bone shortened by disease.

While hip replacement surgery can and usually does restore equal leg lengths, the process for doing so is complex and involves making judgments that can result in leg lengths that are approximately but not exactly equal. Usually, it is possible for a surgeon to make the difference in leg lengths less than half an inch. This small discrepancy is rarely noticed by patients, is probably within the range of normal hip variation, and does not require the use of a shoe lift or alteration in clothing. However, the more complex the deformity of the hip, the more likely the resulting leg lengths will be unequal. Restoring the equality of leg lengths is particularly difficult in revision hip surgery.

A short leg can be safely lengthened by hip surgery up to one and a half inches before important soft tissue structures around the hip, such as nerves and blood vessels, are excessively stretched and damaged. You need to realize that it will be *weeks* or *months* after surgery before you can actually determine how close to equal the length of your legs really are. This is because your pelvis may be tilted after surgery, producing an apparent leg length discrepancy. Swelling of the hip joint, muscle spasm, and muscle weakness can all produce an abnormal, but reversible, pelvic tilt. (See Figure 7-6.)

It will be weeks or months after surgery before you can actually determine how close to equal the length of your legs really are.

Therefore, if your legs appear to be different in length after surgery, particularly if the operated leg appears long, do not panic. It is very likely that this discrepancy is apparent, the result of a pelvic tilt, and will resolve as you continue with the physical therapy that will reduce soft tissue swelling, muscle spasm, and muscle weakness.

Many people who are bothered by the differences in leg lengths during the post-operative recovery period and feel it is hindering their progress of regaining a smooth, even gait consider using a shoe lift. We discourage this, however, because the lift is almost never needed after therapy is completed and the pelvic tilt is corrected. Actually, the use of a lift may prolong the presence of the tilt. Just as important, the use of a lift and the emphasis on leg length measurement that

FIGURE 7-6
Abnormal Pelvic Tilt

The feeling of having a short or long leg following surgery is frequently a result of this form of pelvic tilt. Sometimes the tilt is from a shortening or tightening of the adduction muscles, which physical therapy works to correct.

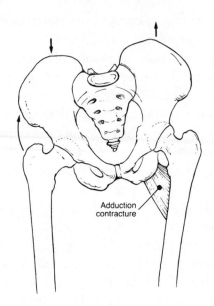

Adduction
contracture

fitting a lift requires may tend to distract you and your physical therapist from the more important rehabilitation issues that you should be dealing with, which are muscle strengthening, muscle stretching, and gait retraining.

First Post-Operative Visit to the Surgeon

Y OUR SURGEON WILL PROBABLY want to see you for the first time three to six weeks after surgery. During this visit, he or she will listen to you carefully, examine you thoroughly, and review your x-rays. Once the surgeon has performed these checks, he or she will be able to explain to you how your recovery is proceeding, how it compares to others, and what you can expect and must do in the next phase of your recovery.

This is an important visit for you, your family, and your surgeon because it is the first opportunity all of you have to discuss what it is like to have a joint replacement. Much of what you learned about joint surgery prior to having the surgery will be clearer, sometimes startlingly so, by that first visit.

PATIENTS OFTEN ARE LESS ACTIVE than they need to be in the first three to four weeks after surgery. Many are worried that they will violate their precautions and something bad will happen, such as dislocating the hip. Some patients, unfortunately, may have taken the first few weeks at home to "feel sick." Although there is a definite period of healing and convalescence that occurs after joint replacement surgery, as there is after all surgeries, the healing after joint surgery almost never prevents people from resuming many of their normal functions, both inside and outside the home. The first office visit is an opportunity for your surgeon to review your activities and therapy of the early post-operative period and modify and extend your exercise program.

How Much Can You Do?

MANY PATIENTS ARE AFRAID THEY will damage their replacement or do something wrong in the first few weeks following surgery. Because the medical and therapy staff often emphasize precautions in the pre-operative and post-operative period, patients naturally focus on them and try hard to avoid activities that might cause something to go wrong. The first post-operative visit provides a good chance to clarify which activities you can and cannot do.

For example, although many patients avoid having sexual intercourse in the first few weeks following surgery, it is permitted after four to six weeks, and you should have been told this in the pre-operative period. Remember to follow the precautions given to you by your surgeon. Most patients of both sexes initially prefer the bottom position, which is more passive and so takes less energy. Be sure to communicate to your partner what is most comfortable for you. Ask your surgeon if you have special concerns.

What Can't You Do?

PATIENTS NORMALLY EXPECT to have a reasonable amount of pain following their surgery. Many find that after a week or two at home, the pain, particularly after hip replacement surgery, is relatively tolerable in comparison to the pre-operative pain from arthritis. However, many patients, especially

Why Are You Still Experiencing Pain?

those who have had total knee replacements, are surprised and unhappy at the amount of pain they feel. Some patients find it very difficult to sleep. Many are worried that their pain is greater than that experienced by others. These patients may be concerned that something is wrong. This issue of pain and all of its related issues must be dealt with clearly and forthrightly, and the first post-operative visit is a good place to discuss them.

Will You Become Dependent on the Pain Medications?

PATIENTS FREQUENTLY FEAR THAT their doctors are more pre-occupied with trying to prevent drug addiction than they are with providing pain relief. The pain following joint replacement surgery, no matter how severe, is at its most severe for the first few weeks and then tapers off by the third month after surgery. This is not enough time for the vast majority of patients to become addicted to the pain medication. Most patients with arthritis, even those who have taken anti-inflammatory agents or analgesics for years, want to stop taking pain medication. That is one reason for undergoing joint replacement surgery in the first place.

In our opinion, concerns about drug addiction in the early post-operative period are not necessary. If a physician is concerned that a patient has a predisposition to drug abuse, he or she should have suspected this in the pre-operative period and should have begun to deal with that issue then. As we discussed in the early in-hospital period, we believe that it is much more likely that you will be under-medicated during your post-operative recovery at home.

Pain control may require the use not only of analgesics, including perhaps narcotics, but also of sleep medication, sedatives, and in selected cases antidepressants. While you may feel that you are not getting enough medication, it may be that you are either not getting the right combination of medications or that you are not taking the medication on the optimum schedule. The first post-operative visit is a good time to review your pain management program.

By the end of the first post-operative visit, you should be ready to change from being a semi-invalid—that is, a patient requiring help from other people and from assistive devices—to a fully independent person. Although the process is different for each patient, you should have a reasonably clear idea of how your recovery is likely to proceed.

Other Follow-Up Visits with Your Surgeon

Y OUR SURGEON WILL PROBABLY want to see you next about three months after surgery, and then again in six to twelve months. Most patients who have undergone primary total joint replacement surgery are independent by three months following surgery. However, the rate of recovery varies widely among patients. Sometimes it is difficult for patients to accept their own recovery schedule, which may take longer than others'. Many patients who have had joint replacement surgery know of someone, often someone older, who has recovered more quickly and has had less pain than they. Chances are very high that your experience, even if prolonged, is not unique or abnormal. Consult your surgeon about any concerns you have.

Conclusion

J OINT REPLACEMENT SURGERY ALLOWS YOU to return to normal activities. In a sense, this surgery forces you to examine clearly what you have and have not been doing in life and why. You cannot start this examination soon enough in your post-operative period. The surgery was done so you could resume, vigorously and without pain, a life you want. The joint replacement surgery relieves the pain from severe arthritis, but it cannot undo habits of behavior and thinking that you have acquired as your painful arthritis has progressed. *You* must do that, and the sooner you start the better.

REHABILITATION:
The IMPORTANCE of PHYSICAL CONDITIONING

S OMETIMES THE BEST REMEDIES are the simplest ones. And the best arthritis cure is not a vitamin, medication, or cream. It is well prescribed and regularly performed exercise. This prescription takes time and requires determination and dedication. Continuous exercise in combination with medication, orthotics, and other interventions as necessary can control the symptoms of most individuals' arthritis. Exercise will rid some persons of their symptoms entirely. What other intervention or cure promises that success?

T HE MEDICAL LITERATURE supporting the benefits of exercise is quite compelling. Regular aerobic exercise improves your cardiovascular conditioning, your sense of well-being, and your lifespan, and it reduces your risk of stroke and heart attack. It also reduces the need for medications for medical conditions such as hypertension, hypercholesterolemia, and diabetes. Persons of all ages experience these benefits.

Positive Effects of Exercise

Reducing the Effects of Arthritis

EXERCISE AS AN ARTHRITIS TREATMENT is becoming increasingly important because it can reverse the deleterious effects of arthritis on the body and influence the effect of arthritis on the joints in particular. Several excellent studies have been published recently on this subject. For example, studies now show that aggressive strength training of the quadriceps and hamstring muscles around the knee reduces the pain and disability that are a consequence of knee arthritis—even in those who have advanced arthritis. Aerobic exercise improves cardiovascular conditioning, helps persons with arthritis control pain with fewer medications, and improves sleep.

Controlling Pain

EXERCISE REDUCES THE PAIN of arthritis by several mechanisms. For instance, increasing the strength and bulk of the quadriceps muscle helps it serve as a more efficient shock absorber for the knee, thus reducing the transmission of force into the knee joint, decreasing pain, and possibly even retarding cartilage deterioration. Exercise improves the range of motion of stiff joints, restoring them to a higher functional level and diminishing pain. Endorphins (pain-reducing hormones produced naturally by the body) are stimulated during aerobic exercise and may help reduce the pain caused by an arthritic hip or knee. These mechanisms combine to maximize the function of the impaired joint, the surrounding joints, and the body overall, leading to a higher level of physical functioning. This is true whether the joint is arthritic or prosthetic.

The Importance of Physical Therapy

FOR A HIP OR KNEE to function normally, it must meet some basic requirements of flexibility and strength. For example, walking without a limp requires the hip to bend at least thirty degrees and to rotate five to eight degrees. A person who wishes to stand up from a squatting position needs significant strength of the quadriceps. If a body cannot meet basic requirements to perform a specific activity, then the body compensates, leading to injury, pain, and incomplete performance.

The common physical limitations seen in arthritic and prosthetic joints can be reduced by appropriate regular exercise. For instance, after hip replacement the hip extensors, abductors, internal rotators, and quadriceps muscles are often disproportionately weak. After knee replacement, the knee is stiff and the hip abductors, hamstrings, and quadriceps are weak. To correct these limitations, specific exercise is required.

However, when patients exercise without supervision they often stretch and strengthen their muscles in the most *expedient* way, sometimes focusing on what is easiest to do rather than on what may be the best for their particular weaknesses. Also, when specific physical impairments exist, the body compensates by using other muscles or adopting an easier position in which to do the exercise. This results in incomplete stretching and strengthening, so despite regular exercise, the patient is not able to attain the desired physical functioning or to reduce pain.

Although there are some common weaknesses that persons with hip and knee arthritis experience, most individuals have limitations that are quite specific to their bodies. For example, one person might have flat feet associated with their knee arthritis, another person might have tight muscles around the artificial hip joint, and yet another person might have especially weak muscles. Thus the best exercise programs are customized to meet each individual's specific needs and then are revised as those needs change. That is why we recommend evaluation by a physiatrist and referral to a physical therapist to design the optimum exercise program. This approach guarantees the best outcome.

The best exercise programs are customized to meet each individual's specific needs and then are revised as those needs change.

Sometimes when starting an exercise program, people develop pain in other joints, such as the back or shoulders. If this occurs, the exercise program must be modified. Pain at or around a joint often is not caused by the deterioration of cartilage seen on x-rays or related to having an artificial joint. Soft tissue disorders, such as bursitis, tendonitis, and muscle overuse injuries, may occur near the joint and cause pain.

These disorders are reversible but are sometimes so chronic that the pain they cause may be mis-attributed as arthritis or normal pain after a joint replacement (despite the fact that there should be none). For example, persons who have prosthetic hips frequently complain about pain at the lateral and anterior thigh. This pain may be dismissed as a routine consequence of a hip replacement or as an early sign of prosthetic loosening. However, sometimes this type of pain is caused from the tightness of a soft tissue structure called the iliotibial band and can be lessened with focused physical therapy and an ongoing home exercise program. A careful physical examination by a physician and an appropriately prescribed physical therapy program can reverse soft tissue pain.

After the physician identifies your physical limitations, which may be subtle, you will be referred to a physical therapist skilled in musculoskeletal therapy who will develop a customized exercise program for you. The physical therapist creates a program that will be effective and address your specific physical needs. In addition, your therapist will supervise you as you perform the exercises to make sure you are doing them correctly.

Dedication and Determination

CONSISTENT DEDICATION TO AN EXERCISE PROGRAM is difficult. You must be determined to succeed. If your goal is to exceed performing your typical daily activities, your devotion to exercise must be even greater because the physical requirements for higher levels of performance—such as those required for long-distance walking, golf, tennis, or running—are more demanding. So although someone with arthritis or a joint replacement may walk without difficulty, he or she might still have problems playing tennis unless the physical skills necessary to perform each aspect of the game have been practiced.

Each activity has its own physical requirements. Tennis and golf require significant hip rotation, while hiking requires extreme knee flexion and substantial quadriceps strength. Still, with regular, appropriate physical exercise, persons who have arthritis or a joint replacement nearly always can attain these higher levels of physical activity.

WE HAVE MANY PATIENTS in our practice who have advanced arthritis or joint replacements yet still enjoy vigorous sports, including skiing, tennis, hiking, and even running. They participate in these activities understanding that researchers still don't know whether this level of exercise helps or hurts their joints. Some surgeons counsel their patients with arthritis or joint replacement to avoid all strenuous—especially weight-bearing—activities.

Effect of Sports on Arthritic and Artificial Joints

The most concern is over sports that involve repetitive pounding or twisting on the limbs. Nearly all surgeons counsel against participation in sports such as football, racquetball, basketball, singles tennis, running, and skiing. Most agree that swimming, biking, golf, doubles tennis, and walking are safe. The fear is that the wrong form of exercise might hasten the deterioration of arthritic joints, cause wear on the plastic liner of a joint replacement, or loosen a joint replacement leading to earlier revision surgery.

In contrast, we believe that bodies properly prepared physically for specific sports should be able to play them as long as each person is knowledgeable about and accepts the potential risks associated with their choice.

Should you perform high levels of exercise? When you are considering this question, understand that the consequences of arthritic and joint replacement patients participating in athletics have not been well defined. One investigator believes that athletics after joint replacement doubles the rate at which the prosthetic joint will wear out. Yet another researcher has published a large study suggesting no effect of activity on joint replacement wear. We just do not have enough evidence yet to respond with a firm yes or no in response to the question. We do know, however, that people who have arthritis and exercise feel much better than their counterparts who do not. Joint replacement patients who exercise also report higher satisfaction with their results than their inactive counterparts. You must weigh the pros and cons about how active you wish to be after surgery.

A Patient's Perspective: Ron

I AM NOW BACK TO PLAYING relatively high-level tennis. It has taken quite an effort to achieve this, but it has been worth the time and energy. I enjoy the game, and thus I feel an element of personal gratification. More importantly, having the goal of being able to play at a reasonable level has been an important motivation for me. However, there are certain risks involved in what I am doing, and thus I cannot recommend that you attempt anything similar to what I have done. What I can do is explain why I have chosen to do what I am doing to help you understand the relevant considerations.

The risks in what I am doing are obvious. As we have seen, a controversy exists about the effects of strenuous activity on the longevity of hip and knee replacements. It is possible that the kind of activity I am doing will cause the replacements to wear out more quickly, thus necessitating revision surgery earlier than otherwise would be the case. This is a real risk, and not a pleasant one. It is also possible, however, that more strenuous activity may not hasten the wearing process, and indeed may delay it. Because exercise strengthens the muscles around the joint, which makes them more efficient shock absorbers, these stronger muscles may actually lessen the rate at which the physical components of the artificial hips wear out. Exercise can also increase bone density, which may be a plus, especially for those with cementless artificial hips, like me.

Still, the jury is out on these questions, and five years from now we may find that I have prematurely worn out the hips to the point where they need replacement again. Why, then, am I doing what I am? I decided that I was willing to take that risk for a number of reasons. I was unwilling at my age to live a sedentary life unless I absolutely had to. Avoiding more strenuous activity now (being sedentary) so that problems don't lead to my being sedentary later—this reasoning did not make sense to me. I did not want to behave as though I were crippled now so that I wouldn't be crippled later. I preferred to take the chance of trying to live the middle part of my life as though I were relatively normal, even if that increased the risk of further surgeries down the road at an earlier time than otherwise would have been the case.

Whether this is sensible or not I really can't say, and I certainly do not recommend that you do likewise simply because I have chosen to do so. The risks, if they materialize, are substantial. Surgery is never fun and always risky. Further, revision surgery may not provide as acceptable a result as you like. So try to think clearly and deeply about these matters before you act.

A Note of Caution

IF YOU HAVE PERSISTENT PAIN or limitations, despite dedication to a customized exercise program, it is possible you have something unusually wrong with your joint. If you have arthritis, you might have torn some cartilage. If you have a joint replacement, the implant itself might have a problem—such as loosening, wear of the plastic liner, heterotopic ossification, a poorly fitted or poorly functioning implant, or other issues. Alternatively, you could be performing your exercises incorrectly without realizing it or you could have a problem elsewhere in your body, such as in your back, that is referring the pain to your leg. When you have persistent pain, you must see your doctor so the cause can be investigated.

How to Exercise

EXERCISE WILL CHANGE YOUR LIFE. But you don't have to wait to have a therapist design a customized program, even though such a program is preferred. You can start now with the exercises shown here.

The exercise program we present is appropriate for those with arthritis, those planning surgery, or those in the later postoperative stages of joint replacement surgery—that is, after the six- to eight-week period of recovery immediately after surgery. *If less than eight weeks have passed since your hip or knee replacement, however, you should not perform these exercises unless you have received approval from your surgeon.* Once you are able to complete this exercise program without difficulty, you are ready for an advanced program. Evaluation by a physiatrist and referral to a physical therapist is necessary to identify your specific needs for an advanced program.

The best exercise format has three phases. The warm-up period usually consists of light aerobic exercise and stretching. This is followed by a period of more rigorous strengthening or aerobic exercises. A brief cool-down period of light stretching and aerobics should complete your workout. A good workout should last from twenty to forty minutes. Exercise in this format reduces injury and maximizes performance.

Alternate days of the strengthening exercise program with an aerobic program.

In addition to the stretching and strengthening exercises that follow, everyone should perform regular aerobic exercise. We usually recommend alternating days of the strengthening home exercise program with an aerobic program, so you perform some form of exercise each day. Aerobic exercises such as walking, bicycling, and swimming increase your heart rate. If you have severe joint disease or have not exercised before, you may wish to begin with walking or a gentle water aerobics program. Begin with five minutes of aerobic exercise and increase the duration each week.

Always check with your doctor before beginning an exercise program. That way any modifications can be made to the program according to any special conditions you may have, such as heart disease or diabetes. Some people require special testing, such as cardiac stress testing, to determine the safest level at which they should exercise. *And if you ever experience chest pain, severe shortness of breath, lightheadedness, or other physical symptoms that worry you during exercise, you should stop immediately and check with your doctor.*

The exercise program we recommend follows. Begin with warm-ups, then proceed to stretching. Follow the stretching with either strengthening exercises or aerobics, on alternating days. Always complete your program with the cool-down period.

Equipment you will need includes a floor mat or a firm surface to lie on, a table or a chair with a firm back, a long length of rubber exercise tubing (obtainable at sports supply stores), a pillow, and a bolster or a rolled up towel.

YOU SHOULD ALWAYS WARM UP before performing the stretching, strengthening, and active aerobic exercise programs. Any light aerobic exercise that slowly moves the muscles is appropriate for warm-ups. For example, walking around the room or using the stationary bike or treadmill are good warm-up exercises. Warm-ups should be followed by the stretching program. The exercise we describe for warm-ups is the stationary bike, but again, any aerobic exercise that involves moving the legs will do.

Warm-Ups

FIGURE 8-1
Stationary Bike

Stationary Bike (See Figure 8-1.) Adjust the bike seat to the correct height. Your knee should be slightly bent when your leg is fully extended on the pedals. Sit on the bike, grip the handles, and pedal with your feet. Pedal briskly for at least 5 minutes.

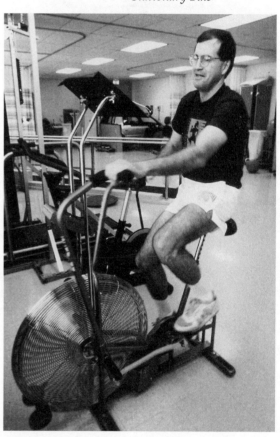

THE STRETCHING PROGRAM FOLLOWS the warm-ups. *Always* stretch before beginning the strengthening or aerobic exercise programs. Stretching will help reduce the chance of injury during either strengthening or aerobic exercise.

Stretching Program

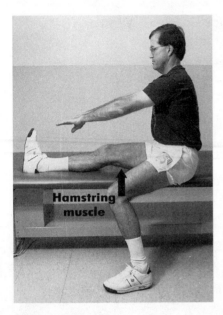

FIGURE 8-2
Hamstring Stretch
(seated)

Hamstring Stretch (See Figure 8-2.) Sit with the left leg off the side of a raised mat, bench, or bed with the foot firmly on the ground. Flex your foot so the toes are pointing toward the ceiling; keep your knee as straight as possible. Lean forward and reach for your toes, keeping your back straight. You should feel the stretch in the back of the right thigh. Hold the position for 6 seconds. Do 10 repetitions. Repeat on your left leg.

Hamstring Stretch (See Figure 8-3.) (a) Lie on your back with your legs straight. Pull the right thigh toward you with your hands.

(b) Now, from the exercise position just described, try to straighten your right knee without moving your hip. You should feel the stretch in the back of your right thigh. Hold the position for 6 seconds. Do 10 repetitions. Repeat on your left leg.

FIGURE 8-3
Hamstring Stretch
(lying down)

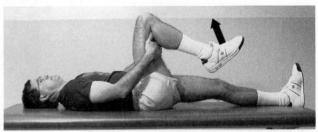

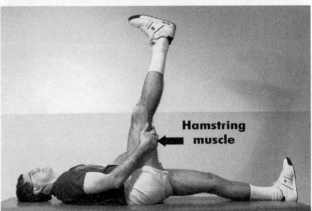

Hip Flexor Stretch (See Figure 8-4.) Lie on your back on a table with your bottom at the edge and your legs dangling. Bring both knees to your chest, with your hands holding the backs of your thighs. Lower the right leg and keep the left knee bent toward your chest. You should feel a stretch on the top of your right thigh. Hold the position for 6 seconds. Do 10 repetitions. Repeat this exercise, lowering your left leg.

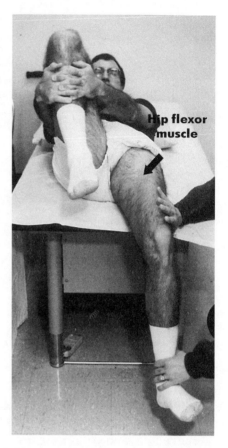

FIGURE 8-4
Hip Flexor Stretch

FIGURE 8-5
Gastrocnemius Stretch

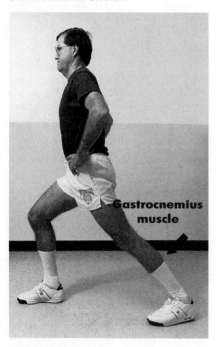

Gastrocnemius Stretch (See Figure 8-5.) With both feet facing forward and hip width apart, step forward with your right foot so your feet are 2–3 feet apart. Keeping your upper body upright, lean forward over your right leg, keep your left knee straight, and keep your left heel on the floor. You should feel a stretch along your left calf (gastroc) muscle. Hold the position for 6 seconds. Do 10 repetitions. Repeat this stretch with your left foot forward and your right foot back.

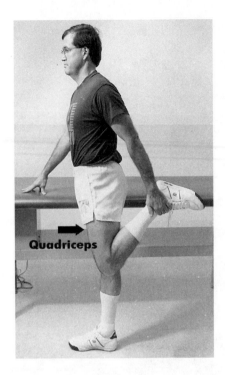

Quadriceps

Quadriceps Stretch (See Figure 8-6.) Standing with your right side next to a table or the back of a stable chair, place your right hand on the table for support and balance, bend your left knee, and hold your left ankle with your left hand. Keep your right knee straight and your body upright. You should feel a stretch along the front of your left thigh (quadriceps). Hold the position for 6 seconds. Do 10 repetitions. Repeat this stretch, facing the opposite direction, with your left leg straight, your right knee bent, and your right ankle held.

FIGURE 8-6
Quadriceps Stretch

FIGURE 8-7
Lateral Hip Stretch

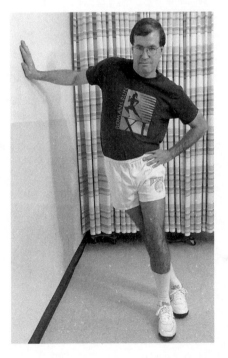

Lateral Hip Stretch (See Figure 8-7.) Standing with your right hand against a wall (fingers toward the ceiling) and your right arm straight and horizontal, cross your right leg behind your left and place your right foot to the outside of your left foot on the floor. Keep both legs straight. Place your left hand on your hip and lean your right hip toward the wall. You should feel a stretch along the outside of your right waist and hip. Hold the position for 6 seconds. Do 10 repetitions. Repeat this stretch, facing the opposite direction, with your left foot behind and to the outside of the right.

Caution: Do not perform this stretch within 8–12 weeks after total hip surgery unless you have your surgeon's approval.

Perform the strengthening program on alternate days from the aerobic exercise program. Remember, start with warm-ups and stretching and finish with cool-down.

Quad Set (See Figure 8-8.) Lie on your back and press the back of the right knee into the mat, tightening the muscle at the front of the thigh. Hold the position for 6 seconds. Do 10 repetitions. Repeat this exercise with your left knee.

Strengthening Exercise Program

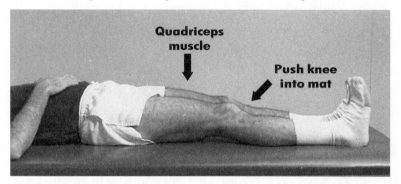

FIGURE 8-8
Quad Set

Terminal Knee Extension (See Figure 8-9.) Lie on your back with a bolster or rolled-up towel under your knees. Straighten your right knee, keeping the back of the knee on the bolster or rolled towel. Hold for 6 seconds and then relax. Do 10 repetitions. Repeat this exercise with your left knee.

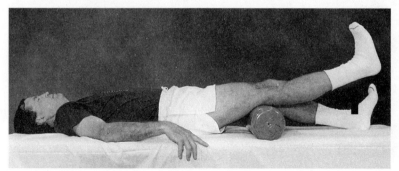

FIGURE 8-9
Terminal Knee Extension

Hamstring Set (See Figure 8-10.) Lie on your back with a bolster or rolled-up towel under your knees. Tighten the muscles behind the right knee as if you were going to bend the knee toward your chest. Then dig your heel into the bed or mat without allowing your right knee to bend. Hold this position for 6 seconds and then relax. Do 10 repetitions. Repeat this exercise with your left knee.

FIGURE 8-10
Hamstring Set

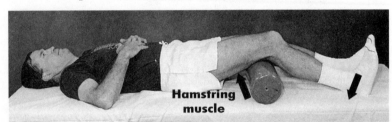

Hip External and Internal Rotation (See Figure 8-11.) Lie on a mat with your feet hip width apart and your toes pointed toward the ceiling. Turn toes out to side. Return to starting position. Hold for 6 seconds. Do 10 repetitions.

Caution: Do not perform this exercise within 8–12 weeks after total hip surgery unless you have your surgeon's approval.

FIGURE 8-11
Hip External and Internal Rotation

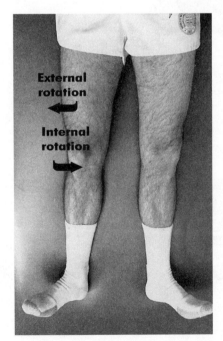

Bridging (See Figure 8-12.) (a) Lie on your back with your knees bent and the soles of your feet placed flat on the mat. (b) Lift your bottom up off the mat, squeezing your buttock muscles. Hold for 6 seconds and then lower your bottom. Do 10 repetitions.

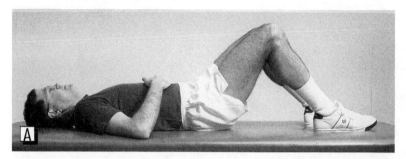

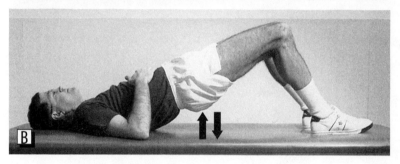

FIGURE 8-12
Bridging

FIGURE 8-13
Side-Lying Hip Abduction

Side-Lying Hip Abduction (See Figure 8-13.) Lie on your side with the bottom knee bent back to support you. Raise the top leg, keeping your knee straight and your toes pointed forward. Do not let the top hip roll backward. Hold 6 seconds. Do 10 repetitions. Roll over and repeat on your other leg.

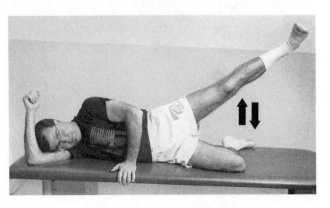

Caution: Do not lie on your operated side within 8–12 weeks after total hip surgery unless you have your surgeon's approval.

Hamstring Curl (See Figure 8-14.) Lie flat with your stomach on the mat and your arms folded under your chin. Bend your left knee, bringing your heel toward your bottom. Do not let your back arch. Hold 6 seconds. Do 10 repetitions. Repeat with your right knee.

FIGURE 8-14
Hamstring Curl

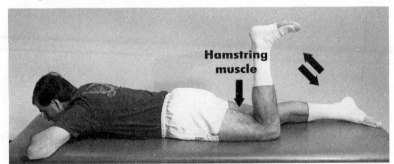

Full Arc Quad (See Figure 8-15.) Sit upright in a chair with your feet flat on the ground. Place a loop of stretch tubing around the chair leg and around your left ankle. Lift and straighten your left leg to stretch the tubing. Hold 6 seconds. Do 10 repetitions. Change position and repeat with your right leg.

FIGURE 8-15
Full Arc Quad

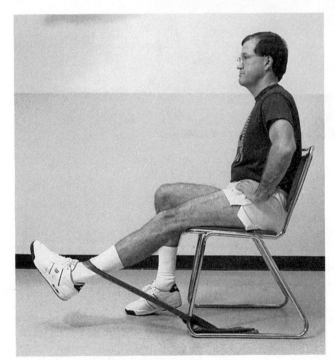

Seated Hip Abduction (See Figure 8-16.) Sit upright with your knees hip width apart. Wrap stretch tubing around your thighs, just above the knees. Spread your legs apart and hold for 6 seconds. Relax. Do 10 repetitions.

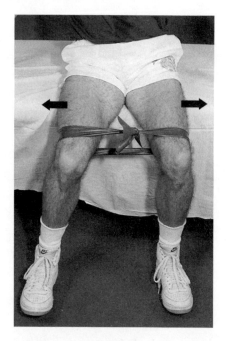

FIGURE 8-16
Seated Hip Abduction

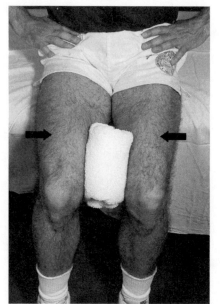

Seated Hip Adduction (See Figure 8-17.) Sit upright and place a folded towel or pillow between your knees. Squeeze the towel between your knees and hold for 6 seconds. Relax. Do 10 repetitions.

FIGURE 8-17
Seated Hip Adduction

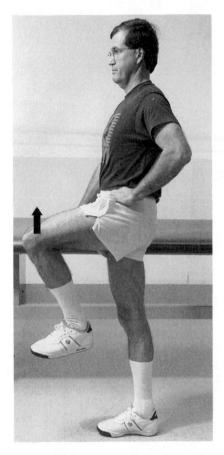

Standing Active Hip Flexion (See Figure 8-18.) Stand in place with one hand resting on a kitchen counter or chair back for support. March in place, raising your knees as high as you can. Do 10 repetitions.

FIGURE 8-18
Standing Active Hip Flexion

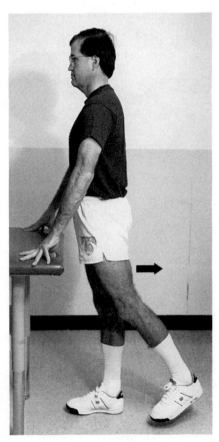

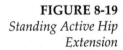

Standing Active Hip Extension (See Figure 8-19.) Stand in place, resting both hands on a table or chair back for support. Squeeze your buttock muscles. With your knee straight, raise your left leg behind you as high as you can. Keep your trunk upright. Hold 6 seconds. Do 10 repetitions. Repeat with your right leg.

FIGURE 8-19
Standing Active Hip Extension

Standing Active Knee Flexion (See Figure 8-20.) Stand in place, resting both hands on a table or chair back for support. Raise your left leg as high as you can, bending it back at the knee toward your bottom. Hold 6 seconds. Do 10 repetitions. Repeat with your right leg.

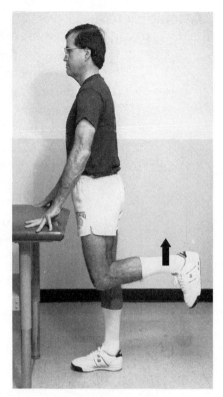

FIGURE 8-20
*Standing Active
Knee Flexion*

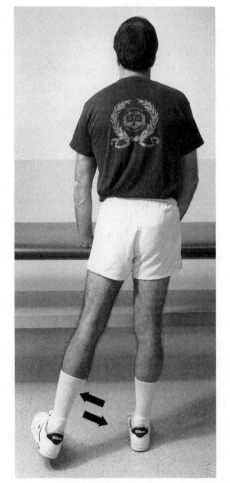

21. Standing Active Hip Abduction (See Figure 8-21.) Stand in place and rest both hands on a table or chair back for support. Raise your left leg to the side as high as you can without leaning over. Keep your knee straight and your trunk upright. Hold 6 seconds. Do 10 repetitions. Repeat the exercise with your right leg.

FIGURE 8-21
*Standing Active
Hip Abduction*

Aerobic Exercise Program

WALKING IS EXCELLENT AEROBIC EXERCISE. Other effective aerobic exercises include bicycling, swimming, rowing, and aerobic dance. Any exercise that raises your heart rate will be effective. The ultimate goal to set for yourself is to perform your aerobic exercise for 30 minutes three to four times per week. Begin with 5 minutes of exercise and add 5 minutes per week until you reach 30 minutes per session. Don't skip aerobic exercise!

For aerobic exercise to be effective, you must attain your *target heart rate* during exercise. Your target heart rate is roughly calculated by subtracting your age from the number 220 and multiplying that by .8 if you are physically healthy, and .6 if you have never exercised or have other medical conditions. You can measure your heart rate by taking your pulse for 15 seconds and multiplying that number by 4. (Place your fingertips on your wrist and count the beats.) For example, if you are sixty years old and have never exercised, your target heart rate is 220 minus 60 equals 160; 160 times .6 equals 96. You should have a pulse of at least 96 during exercise.

Cool-Down

THE COOL-DOWN PERIOD SHOULD LAST 3 to 5 minutes. We prefer active cool-down exercises (such as walking) to stretching for cool-down. This may be different from other exercise programs you have been taught. Walk slowly around the room or on the treadmill, or you may slowly pedal the stationary bicycle. This cool-down exercise is meant to gradually ease your heart and muscles back to their resting state.

A Patient's Perspective: Ron

I LEARNED SEVERAL LESSONS from the surgical and rehabilitation experience on my left hip that I subsequently applied to my right hip. Most importantly, if I wanted to have a hip that functioned normally and without pain, I had to take responsibility and initiative to achieve that goal.

After the operation on my left hip, I followed the conventional rehabilitation regime prescribed by most orthopedic surgeons and physical therapists. I received physical therapy for about six weeks.

The exercises and physical therapy were designed to get me walking comfortably without support and without a limp, which they succeeded in doing very well. I was walking without support or pain six weeks after the operation. I was able to drive even earlier. I was able to return to a more or less normal daily routine at about eight weeks. However, I did not have a normal hip. It felt stiff when I tried to do certain things, like drying my lower leg after a shower, or after sitting for more than half an hour. As I became increasingly active, I found numerous other movements that I could not do easily, because of either pain or weakness in my hip.

As far as I could tell, there was no pattern to what I could and could not do easily. I discovered at a cocktail party, for example, that I could not bend down to pick up an hors d'oeuvre from a coffee table if I was standing with my left foot forward. My hip and leg were too weak. Getting out of bed on the left side of the bed one morning, I discovered that when my left leg was free of the bed I could not hold up my lower leg. It rotated from the knee downward, almost in a free fall. I also discovered that, lying on my stomach with my knees bent at a ninety degree angle so that my feet faced the ceiling, I could not roll to the left to get onto my side; if I tried to do so, I experienced intense pain in my thigh. I could not easily walk up and down stairs. Walking up stairs, I lurched; and walking down stairs, I fell as much as strode. I also had some of what I call free-standing pain. Even though the hip was tremendously improved in terms of comfort, nonetheless I had some pain that just seemed to come and go and was not associated with any activity or movement. The best example of this was that I had the thigh pain that so many hip recipients complain about.

None of this pain or weakness felt to me as though the joint itself were to blame; all of it felt like muscular limitations. Dissatisfied with my physical condition, I decided to try to improve it. I acted on this decision in two different ways. First, I decided to increase the general strength and conditioning of my legs through aerobic exercise. I began by increasing my use of a stationary bicycle. I had been using a stationary bicycle since about the fourth week following surgery, and now I got serious about it. About the eighth week following surgery, I began using a treadmill, first doing just level walking, and later walking up an incline. After about three months, my legs felt strong enough for a greater challenge,

Lessons Learned After My First Joint Replacement

My Own Initiative

and I moved up to a stair-stepper. By the time I quit using the stair-stepper (about a year later), I was able to go for more than a half hour at the next to highest level.

My experience with aerobic exercise was quite consistent: my general conditioning continually improved. Although each time I moved to a new activity I had difficulty getting started, I soon was able to progress to higher levels of difficulty. My body—my hip in particular—was more or less functioning normally. As I improved my general conditioning, I felt considerably better, and getting around in life became easier. But the pain I experienced in the motions mentioned above did not go away; it lessened but did not disappear.

Consequently, I decided to add a second strategy to my conditioning effort. For every pain or weakness that I experienced, I constructed an exercise to work the relevant muscles, usually one that simply mimicked the uncomfortable motion, and added it to David's general exercise regime, which I continued to do (adding weights to my ankles as I went along).

Because of the progress I had made on my left hip, David and I decided that for my right hip I should get more serious physical therapy than I had had after the first operation. Fortunately, I met Vicky Brander, who came to direct my physical therapy. She viewed me not as some special case, but instead as a person who wished to regain normal hip function, no different from anybody else who had muscular deficits. She immediately saw that, *while I had done some things right, I had done others wrong, or neglected them entirely.* In brief, I had overdeveloped some muscles, underdeveloped others, and generally emphasized strength almost to the exclusion of flexibility. She put me on a rehabilitation program designed to completely rehabilitate my right hip, which had just been operated on, and also to fix certain long-standing problems in my left leg and hip. With the help of very talented physical therapists, I was astounded with the results. After nine weeks, all the discomfort in my left hip and leg had been eliminated, I had no analogous discomfort on my right side, the range of motion of the right side was soon normal, and the strength on both sides now was at or beyond the normal range in all directions.

Applying Those Lessons

Why had the rehabilitation of my right hip gone so well, and how were Vicky and the physical therapists able to straighten out the problems of my left side? There are three crucial variables.

First, I knew what to do before and after surgery. Because I had already gone through surgery and rehabilitation on my left hip, I knew what to expect for my right hip, what to hope for from the surgery, and what to do. In particular, immediately upon waking following surgery, I began rehabilitation by contracting and then relaxing all the leg and hip muscles I could while lying in my hospital bed. During the week in the hospital, I spent all the energy I could muster on rehabilitation, and again, I was very pleased with the results. I walked the first day following surgery with a walker, and sat up for a number of hours. From the second day forward, I spent most of my waking hours out of bed (many of them exercising). By the third day, I could get in and out of bed by myself and began walking with crutches. I walked with crutches for two weeks, one week more with one crutch, and one week with a cane. By the fifth week following surgery, I could walk without support and without a limp or pain. Virtually all this resulted from my beginning to work on the muscles as soon as I awoke, and from continuing to work diligently on them without letup.

Second, I worked hard to maintain physical fitness long after the surgery. Since my first operation I have been working reasonably diligently on both of my legs and hips. Even though my own program had its limits, as I described above, it also developed a number of the muscles quite well. Going into my second operation, a number of the muscles were very strong and needed only to recover from the trauma of the operation itself, which they did rather quickly. That meant that the range of serious problems was small and could be isolated quickly, so I could concentrate my efforts on them.

Third, my therapists and I kept full recovery as the goal. Ever since Vicky took control of my rehabilitation I have been receiving superb physical therapy advice, governed by the principle that we expected to achieve full recovery. This has made a world of difference. Following my first operation, I received the standard "get 'em up and walking easily" kind of physical therapy. The therapist accomplished her appointed task, and from then on I was on my own. But walking comfortably and having normal hips are quite different matters. Vicky and my physical therapists have kept normal hips as my goal, and have the knowledge and skill to assist me in obtaining it. I have been astounded with the difference from the rehabilitation for my first hip replacement.

For all these reasons, I am now blessed with essentially normal hips for the first time in over thirty years. It has taken a lot of work, but I have learned that it can be done. All it takes is will and good advice.

Sport-Specific Training

STRENGTH AND FLEXIBILITY ARE IMPORTANT components of any functional activity, but having these skills does not necessarily mean you will be able to return to your desired activity level easily. You may have developed alternative ways of performing sport-specific activities to compensate for your physical limitations. These compensation strategies put you at risk for injuries, such as muscle strains, tendonitis, bursitis, and others. You and your physician must determine the specific physical requirements of your sport and whether or not you can meet those requirements.

Once your body is physically prepared to return to a sport, with adequate strength, flexibility, and conditioning, you often have to relearn how to perform the sport correctly. A physical therapist is essential for this phase of recovery. Your physical therapist will be able to help you break down your specific skill needs and then devise exercises to help you meet those needs.

For example, a golf swing requires a significant amount of hip rotation from one direction to the other. A common substitution pattern observed in golfers with hip osteoarthritis is excessive rotation at the spine during the swing, to make up for their lack of hip rotation. This pattern often leads to low back pain as well as a gradual deterioration in the quality of the swing. The physical therapist can analyze the golfer during swing to assess whether an adequate amount of hip rotation exists, whether the hip musculature is strong enough, and whether the hip muscles are working together in a timely and coordinated manner to allow the correct technique to occur.

The physical therapist can then prescribe exercises based on the problem identified. Stretching is prescribed if flexibility is inadequate, position-specific strengthening is recommended if strength is the problem, and coordination-timing drills at the driving range might be included if coordination is limited. Then, once the specific problem areas are resolved, you practice the sport in its specific context. That is, the golfer has to practice on the uneven terrain of the golf course, the tennis player has to practice in the fast-paced situation of a game, the person taking walks in the city has to practice navigating through crowds and traffic.

A gradual and systematic return to higher level activity will ensure a safe and successful return to sport activities.

Do not expect to pick up where you left off prior to your arthritic symptoms or surgery. A gradual and systematic return to higher level activity will ensure a safe and successful return to sport activities.

Conclusion

OF COURSE, EACH PERSON who has osteoarthritis of the hips or knees has distinct needs. In every case the general program described in this chapter should be modified to fit those needs, and to do so requires a skilled physiatrist or physical therapist. Also, in the early stages of your recovery (the first three or four months), much of what needs to be done cannot be done safely on your own. To safely reach your full potential, work closely with a physical therapist.

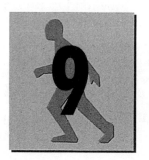

LIVING with an IMPLANT

ONE OF THE MOST DIFFICULT feelings to express to joint replacement patients is what it really feels like to live with an artificial implant. Patients are told before the operation what they will and will not be allowed to do. They are also informed about complications that can occur after the procedure is performed. Yet it is hard to imagine what it will be like having a foreign device in your body for ten, twenty, or perhaps forty years. Will you feel it? If the implant comes loose or starts to wear out, will you sense it? What happens if you overdo it, or fall, or twist a funny way? If your arthritic hip or knee is quite painful, you may think these things don't matter as long as the operation eliminates the pain. But these things will matter to you as soon as you have recovered from the operation.

What It Feels Like

W**E DRAW HERE UPON** Ron's experiences with his total hip replacements to provide you with a sense of what it is like to live with a total joint replacement. Recall that he had received his left hip implant in 1988 and his right one in 1993. In 1995, however, Ron fell and fractured his femur over the stem of the left hip prosthesis. Then, in 1997, Ron underwent a revision of his left hip replacement. Thus, through his experiences we are able to provide you with a sense of what you will feel like once your total joint is functioning as you anticipated, what you might experience if you have a significant complication associated with your implant, and what you might anticipate if you must ever confront the prospect of revision surgery on your total joint replacement.

A Patient's Perspective: Ron

I have since learned how vital rehabilitation is to feeling right.

L**IVING WITH AN IMPLANT** has both a physical and a psychological dimension. I begin with the physical side because that is the simplest. Artificial hips, as far as I can tell, create no abnormal or odd sensations. I don't feel an alien presence within my joints, nor do I detect any sliding or rubbing. My hips do not feel numb, and the attached prosthesis feels no different to me from the rest of my skeletal structure.

However, had I been asked *prior* to my second operation what it was like to have an artificial hip, I would have given a somewhat different answer. I would have said that it does not feel odd in any way, but I would also have said that it is a bit stiffer than a normal hip, and that from time to time it is a little uncomfortable. I would have hastened to add that, even at its worst, it is ten times better than the hip it replaced. But I would not have given it a one hundred percent approval rating. I have since learned how vital rehabilitation is to feeling right.

Psychologically, I am aware of the possible ways I might damage my implants. So I take certain precautions like not playing basketball, jogging on hard surfaces, or going downhill skiing. I no longer dwell on the fact that I have artificial hips or their risks; I feel no omnipresent sense of risk.

If anything, my self-concept now is that of an unimpaired person. Prior to the surgeries, I was constantly aware of my physical limitations, which affected my affairs with those around me. I was in pain and could not do normal tasks easily, or sometimes at all. This was obvious to anyone who saw me move, and I knew that it was. There was no natural end to this condition; it was not going to go away. I observed myself transforming from a strong, athletic person into a seriously impaired individual with no great hope of returning to the person I had been. All this changed dramatically following my surgeries. I regained mobility and strength, and felt like I had reason to hope. Normal day-to-day tasks that previously had been difficult reverted to normal day-to-day tasks. I could even think of playing tennis again, and the pain I had once felt when lying in bed with my wife was gone. I no longer wondered what everybody else was thinking as I limped around.

So my story really is a rosy one. In comparison to both my physical and psychological states prior to surgery, my present states are infinitely improved. I am so much better off than I was that I find it difficult to explain. I am aware of the risks I face and the work I must continue to do to maintain my strength and flexibility, but these issues seem to me within the range of normal human concerns.

Ron's first hip replacement relieved him of most of his pain and allowed him to return to a very high level of function. But for some time it did not feel as good as he hoped it would or thought it should. This may happen to you. There are a number of reasons for this. Some of these may be related to the total joint implant, and some may be related to the way the recovery, including rehabilitation, has occurred. In Ron's case, both implant issues and rehabilitation factors influenced what it was like for him to live with his artificial hips.

Problems That Can Cause Pain

A Patient's Perspective: Ron

T HE KEY TO PROPERLY IMPLANTED hips feeling normal is rehabilitation, and you have to take responsibility for it yourself. Regrettably, your orthopedist may not see that you get adequate physical therapy. For all my high regard for David, my one minor complaint is that he disregarded certain symptoms that should have gotten me to Vicky a year or two earlier. An example is the knee pain I had been complaining about, off and on, for over two years. David, being an orthopedist, would take x-rays, which showed that my knees were completely normal. From his perspective, there was nothing wrong with my knees, and anyway a little knee pain in someone who had been through what I had been through, and who was now able to do what I was able to do, was of no great significance.

However, my knee continued to hurt from time to time, as did my thigh and groin. We now know that this is because of muscular deficiencies that have since been corrected through physical therapy. Your hip can feel completely normal too. It will do so, however, only if you rehabilitate it correctly and completely, and you have to take responsibility for doing so. Although I chide David for not paying enough attention to my complaints, in fact the error lay with me. I should have pursued the matter further and taken appropriate action.

Alerting the Orthopedist to Your Discomfort

I T IS IMPORTANT FOR YOU to realize that the orthopedist who performed your replacement will be concerned, possibly even preoccupied, by issues related to the implants or the technique used to put them in. These preoccupations may cause your surgeon to be inappropriately cautious or perhaps—as I, David, was with Ron—not as creative as I should have been with regard to his therapy program. *If your joint replacement is not feeling quite as well as you expected, you can help focus your orthopedist's attention if you convey as clearly and persistently as possible, as Ron did, your desire to do whatever is necessary and appropriate to feel the way you know a successful joint replacement should.*

Such an approach, indicating your awareness that a successful joint replacement requires effort on your part as well as the surgeon's, may help your orthopedist overcome a somewhat cautious approach to treating your discomfort. By expressing to your orthopedist that you realize he or she alone is not responsible for your discomfort, you will help focus attention on things (such as therapy or drug modification) that are likely to make you feel better.

THE MOST FREQUENT CAUSE of incomplete pain relief after a total joint replacement is inadequate rehabilitation. Physicians often underestimate the role rehabilitation plays in *relieving pain* after a total joint replacement. Physicians and therapists are accustomed to thinking of physical therapy as a way of improving function and strength. In their minds, more therapy may be associated with the production of pain, not its relief.

Yet, these same individuals regularly recommend therapy for patients who have pain associated with a wide variety of musculoskeletal ailments. These physicians and therapists realize that each individual's therapy requirements are unique and depend, among other things, upon the level of function to which a patient wishes to return. Patients who have had an injury and wish to return to pain-free, high-performance athletics will require more therapy than patients wishing to return to less vigorous activities. The same is true of total joint surgery patients like Ron who wish to return to high-level athletics. Patients who wish to be athletic require more intensive and specifically focused physical therapy than the average patient who has had a joint replacement.

However, you should not be misled by the uniqueness of Ron's situation. Although he required relatively intensive therapy to return to pain-free tennis, many patients who simply wish to return to pain-free, unlimited walking also often require more therapy than they receive. Chances are that, if you are not quite completely comfortable six to nine weeks after your total joint surgery, you need more, not less, therapy.

Inadequate Rehabilitation

The most frequent cause of incomplete pain relief after a total joint replacement is inadequate rehabilitation.

Re-Injury

WHEN RON FELL IN 1995 and fractured his left femur, the leg did not need a cast because it was stable. The fracture was in the bone around the prosthesis, so the prosthesis held the bone in place. Figure 9-1 is the x-ray showing the break.

FIGURE 9-1
Left Hip Fracture

In 1995 Ron fell and broke his left femur near the upper end of his implant.

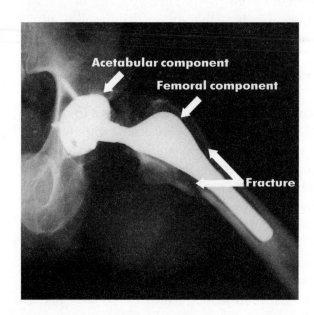

A Patient's Perspective: Ron

"SHOULD I HAPPEN TO BREAK a femur, I will have a real mess on my hands." Talk about words coming back to haunt you! This is exactly what happened. I was ice skating in December 1995 with my boys, Michael and Conor, who were just learning to skate and play ice hockey. I felt quite good, comfortable enough with my new hips to be on ice skates, and really did not think it a big deal. The boys were fooling around with some hockey sticks and pucks. A puck went past me on my left, so I pivoted to the left, just to watch it go by. My skates slipped out from under me, and I landed full force on my left thigh.

It hurt, but I was able to get up and limp off the ice. I sat down and almost passed out. I tried to take a few steps. It was excruciating to put weight on my left leg, but the leg did not feel broken. I thought I knew this because I had experienced a broken femur as a teenager. It just hurt incredibly, but I thought maybe this was just a deep bruise or a hip pointer. I could move, and my leg was not flopping around.

The next day saw no improvement, and every movement was agonizing. I went to David's office for an x-ray, which showed I had fractured my femur. The next five months of my life were not fun. For the first month or so following the break, I was in serious discomfort. This began to reduce, but it still took approximately three months before I was able to walk without crutches, and another month before I gave up a cane. During this time I was receiving therapy prescribed by Vicky and performed by a physical therapist. The good news is that the bone did heal enough to allow me to play tennis again in the summer of 1995 and 1996. The bad news is that, notwithstanding a prodigious effort, it never was truly comfortable again.

What Is the Likelihood of Fracture or Dislocation?

THE MAJORITY OF FALLS PRODUCING pain or episodes of acute swelling and pain are, in fact, usually not serious. Pain around a joint replacement, particularly after a fall or unusual period of activity, is common. As time passes, you will learn, as Ron did, to distinguish this type of discomfort from the pain associated with a serious problem. Until you develop confidence in your ability to distinguish the signs and symptoms of pain associated with a serious problem from those associated with vigorous everyday living, consult your orthopedist when something out of the ordinary occurs.

Although Ron's experience, fortunately, is rare, it does highlight a number of issues important to patients living with a total joint implant. The first is that dramatic, sudden things can happen to artificial joints that are less likely to occur in joints that have not been replaced. The bone around the implants can fracture, and artificial joints can dislocate.

You may wonder how likely it is for these things to occur once you have recovered from surgery. You may also wonder if you will constantly be thinking about the possibility of catastrophic events occurring to your replaced joints. In fact, events such as fractures or dislocation are extremely rare once recovery from surgery is complete, which is usually in about three months. For such mishaps to occur, a significant fall (as in Ron's case) has to take place, or a significant focus of untreated infection has to exist. Thus, *if you are reasonably prudent and watchful, you do not have to fear that a catastrophic event will occur to your artificial joint.* Most surgeons, therefore, suggest that patients avoid activities (such as uncontrolled downhill skiing) that can cause a significant fall.

Virtually all patients stop thinking, as Ron did, about whether the activities they have returned to will produce a catastrophic failure of their implant. You will quickly become comfortable with a level of activity that you are confident is safe. The important thing is to recognize what it is you are safely capable of doing, with or without a joint replacement.

Does a Fracture around an Implant Require Surgery?

WHEN A FEMUR BREAKS in a leg with an artificial hip, surgery is frequently the only option. If the break occurs below the prosthesis, the bone almost always has to be repaired surgically. If it breaks around the prosthesis and if the prosthesis is loose, the implant usually must be replaced to stably fix the fracture. If the prosthesis is the cemented variety, this is always the case. But Ron's case was unusual. The prosthesis had held the pieces of bone together and had not greatly dislodged from the femur. Because it was a bony fixation implant, the bone would possibly grow back into the prosthesis. We thus decided to wait and see what happened. We did not cast the leg because the bone seemed stable. So began a three-month period on crutches while we waited to see what the bone would do.

Will the Implant Need to Be Replaced?

YOU MAY WONDER IF YOUR IMPLANT will have to be removed or exchanged if a catastrophic event, such as a fracture or dislocation, occurs. The response to this concern may be complicated, for it depends upon many factors. However, in general, if your implant was correctly aligned and well fixed *before* the catastrophic event, the chances are good that it will be left in place while the specific event (such as a fracture) is treated.

Because this is the case, it is important that *if you believe you may have developed a problem with your artificial joint, you should report it promptly to your surgeon.* Obviously, breaking a femur, as Ron did, should not be hard to recognize. Yet even in Ron's case, hoping as he was that he had just bruised his hip and not injured his implants (and being accustomed over the years to painful falls), he waited a bit before seeking help.

It never hurts to check things out if you think something is wrong. Sometimes getting help quickly may save the implant or avoid a large operation. For example, if Ron's fracture, which was essentially undisplaced, had become very mal-aligned, he would have needed an operation to correct the alignment (and probably replace the implant).

After Re-Injury, Will the Joint Be Pain Free Again?

YOU MAY WONDER if you will regain the same level of pain relief and function after a catastrophic event. Will a total hip that has dislocated ever be pain free? Will you ever stop worrying that such a thing could happen again? Obviously there cannot be a single, simple answer to such a concern, for many factors influence the final level of pain and function of an injured total joint replacement. However, one rule applies to the overwhelming majority of such cases. *If the joint replacement was well fixed, well aligned, and pain free before the event, the chances are very good that it will be that way again, once the problem has been corrected.* However, it will take time to heal, more time than a normal joint without a replacement. And it will take significant effort on your part, an effort as great or greater than that which you exerted during your recovery from the original surgery.

Joints with replacements should be thought of in the same way as joints with a mild amount of arthritis. Such joints can and usually do function at a very high level without pain. Remember, for many years Ron played very active tennis on a hip with a substantial degree of arthritis. However, when such joints undergo a significant injury, they hurt more and recover more slowly than joints that are completely normal. The less arthritis in the injured joint, the faster and more complete the recovery. Likewise, the better the fixation and alignment of the implants, the faster and more complete the recovery of an injured replacement. Just as patients with a mildly arthritic joint (often one they thought was completely normal, because it never hurt) are surprised at the time and effort it takes to recover completely, patients with pain-free total joint replacements are surprised and frustrated at how long it takes and how much work is involved to return to pre-injury function.

Because patients are understandably worried that the joint replacement has been damaged, they often interpret prolonged pain after a catastrophic event as a sign that something is wrong. Some patients' well-fixed, well-aligned implants remain sore for almost a year after a single event, such as a dislocation. The most important thing to remember is that in a very large majority of cases, injuries to joint replacements that are well-aligned and well-fixed rarely jeopardize that fixation, and almost never accelerate a process of wear or failure of the implant system.

Revision (Replacement) Surgery

ALTHOUGH ALL PATIENTS WHO UNDERGO joint replacement surgery worry about the prospect of having to have their implants replaced or revised, the actual percentage of patients who require a revision is very small. If you are in your mid-sixties or older and undergo total joint surgery, you have a very high likelihood of living the rest of your life without having to face such surgery. However, if you are younger, like Ron, you are more likely to require a revision of your implant.

You can not only help reduce the likelihood of needing a revision, you can also influence the extent and seriousness of the surgery, if it is necessary, by being aware of the issues related to the revision of replacement implants.

Common Causes

ALTHOUGH TOTAL JOINT IMPLANTS MAY need to be revised for many reasons (and the most common reasons for hip replacement revisions are not the same as those for knee replacement revisions), the two reasons of most concern to all hip or knee patients are wear of the materials and implant loosening. If you are likely to have your implant for more than ten to fifteen years, you may need to confront one or both of these causes for revision surgery. Additional reasons include bone loss and characteristics of the patient.

Wear of the implant materials, especially the plastic, in total hip implants produces particles that float around in the hip joint. These particles can lodge themselves between the implants and the bone, if there is space between them. In the case of Ron's hip, the incompletely coated femoral implant left some areas of space between implant and bone into which the plastic particles could migrate. When plastic particles get near bone, they prompt a chemical reaction that causes bone to dissolve. As the bone dissolves, the implant becomes less well-fixed to bone. As the implant's fixation to bone decreases, the hip becomes painful, especially during significant activity. Thus, Ron had specific implant-related issues that might have been the source of his pain. *Wear of the Implant*

These implant issues (plastic wear and implant fixation) are of concern whether the components are uncemented, as in Ron's case, or cemented. They are, in fact, the issues that orthopedists tend to focus on as they follow patients with joint replacements.

As we begin to observe the results of total joint implants that have been in hips for fifteen to twenty years, it is becoming clear that wear of the implants is the factor that is most likely to determine the lifespan of total joint implants. Wear causes the revision of total joint components in two ways: by leading to loosening of the implants and by producing osteolysis.

To function without pain, all total joint implants must be well-fixed to the bone, whether with or without cement. If the fixation is not secure, a total joint implant moves and thereby causes pain. If a cemented implant was not well fixed to bone at the time of the original joint replacement, or if an *Loosening of the Implant* uncemented implant does not become well-fixed to bone in the first few months after the original joint replacement, then progressive loosening of the implant is likely to occur relatively quickly (within one to four years after surgery). However, if the original implants are well-fixed to bone, then loosening may not occur for ten to twenty years, if at all.

Osteolysis
(Bone Loss)

Debris particles from a worn implant also cause the secretion of a number of chemicals that are capable of producing extensive bone loss. This bone loss is called *osteolysis*. Entire segments of bone can dissolve because of these chemicals. Osteolysis is the most serious long-term undesirable effect of total joint implants. Osteolysis can lead to implant revision in at least two ways. It can cause the implants to come loose in the bone. It can also cause the bone itself to become so weakened that worn implants need to be exchanged to prevent the remaining bone from dissolving further.

Because loose total joint implants are usually painful, patients almost always seek medical attention for this pain before the implants become so loose that they threaten the integrity of the bone. However, osteolysis may occur to quite an extent without producing symptoms. This process does not usually begin in any significant degree for six to ten years after a total joint replacement.

Because a successful total joint revision requires an adequate amount of bone for implant fixation, it is important that *if you have had a total joint replacement for more than eight to ten years, you should see your orthopedist regularly, even if you have no symptoms.* Ron's experience is a good illustration of the interaction between implant loosening and wear and their impact on a patient's symptoms. Ron had x-ray evidence of plastic wear, mostly in his femur, for some time before his revision. Yet he remained reasonably comfortable until his femoral component loosened. He also had x-ray evidence of wear behind his acetabular component. However, this component remained firmly fixed to bone and never caused symptoms of any kind. (See Figure 9-2.)

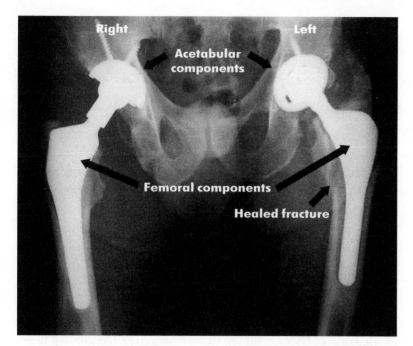

FIGURE 9-2
Fracture Healed,
Pre-Revision

The bone was able
to heal within the
implant, but the
component became
unstable. The hip never
felt as comfortable as it
had before his fall.
Note the bone spurs
above the left femoral
component.

Many factors related to the characteristics of patients with total joint replacements may influence the wear and loosening of implants. We have discussed these in earlier chapters. Your weight, the types of activities you engage in, and the quality of your bone probably all affect the durability of fixation of a total joint implant. Because the exact relationship of these patient-related factors to loosening is not currently known, we have suggested throughout this book that reasonableness is probably the most prudent course.

Thus, keeping your weight within twenty percent of the desired weight for your overall size and age, limiting your activities to sports that are not high impact, and following an exercise, diet, and drug program that minimizes the likelihood of osteoporosis (including calcium, vitamin D, and possibly estrogens and drugs that promote increased bone mineral density) are most likely to help ensure secure fixation of your implant. Overdoing any of these precautions (such as weighing less than your desired weight, being inactive, or

Characteristics of
the Patient

taking excessive amounts of vitamin D and calcium) is unlikely to add longevity to your implant and may even jeopardize its fixation. Being too thin or too inactive may make your muscles weak and osteoporosis more likely and thus may adversely affect fixation of your implant.

An Overview of Revision Surgery

ALTHOUGH THE PREPARATION FOR and the performance of a revision total joint replacement are very similar to those for a primary joint replacement, there are a few critical differences. *First*, the revision procedure is very likely to be more complex and longer than the primary surgery, so the pre-operative preparation may be more involved. A joint aspiration may be necessary to ensure that there is no infection present. This procedure is very much like a joint injection and can usually be carried out in the surgeon's office with local anesthesia. A revision procedure also requires more blood than a primary procedure. *Second*, because patients are older than they were at the time of their primary procedure, they frequently need a more extensive pre-operative medical examination. *Finally*, and most importantly, the risks of complications (including infection, fracture, dislocation, and blood clotting) and the period of recovery are greater in revision surgery than in primary surgery.

Revision surgery often requires that lost bone material be replaced. This can be a complex undertaking. Bone graft, obtained either from the patient or from a bone bank, may be needed to replace lost bone. Special implants that take up the space formerly occupied by bone may need to be used. The bone graft must be firmly attached to the remaining bone so it can become incorporated into the host bone. Plates, rods, and wires may be needed to achieve this firm attachment. Similarly, the special implants must be rigidly fixed to the remaining bone.

Revision implants, like primary implants, may be cemented or uncemented. However, the shapes of these devices are usually different in important respects from primary implants. For example, the lengths of the stems which insert into bone may be longer, or the porous coating may be more extensive. (See Figure 9-3, which shows Ron's revision implant.) In fact, because the exact requirements of many revision procedures cannot be exactly predicted prior to the surgery, it is frequently necessary to have a wide variety of bone grafting options and implant choices available in the operating room during the performance of a revision total joint procedure.

Because the revision procedures are more complex, it is important not only that they be performed by a surgeon who is familiar with the requirements of this type of surgery, but also that they be carried out at hospitals properly equipped for such cases. Removing the original implants and cement

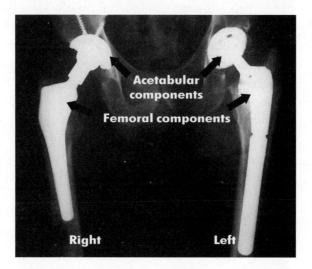

FIGURE 9-3
Post-Revision of Left Hip

By 1996 Ron's left hip discomfort had increased, and revision surgery was performed. The femoral component, which was loose, was replaced with a longer implant.

may require special equipment not present at all hospitals. Monitoring parts of the procedure with fluoroscopic x-rays may be necessary, and this necessary equipment must be available in the hospital's operating room. The equipment used for revisions is extensive and complex and should be familiar to the operating room personnel. Peri-operative management may require special monitoring capabilities. Thus, it is not uncommon that a patient who has had a primary total joint replacement done well by one surgeon undergo a revision many years later by a different surgeon at a different hospital.

Rehabilitation Care after Revision Surgery

THE POST-OPERATIVE CARE OF PATIENTS who have undergone revision joint replacements generally is similar to that following a primary replacement, but may vary in the particulars. For example, because revision total hip replacements are more likely to dislocate than primary replacements, hip precautions may be enforced for a longer period of time. Special braces may even be used to prevent dislocations. Depending on the extent and type of the procedure, mobilization and rehabilitation may differ significantly between primary and revision procedures. If bone grafting was extensive, weight-bearing may be restricted for a substantial period of time, and the use of assistive devices such as crutches may be significantly prolonged. Muscle rehabilitation invariably takes significantly longer after a revision procedure than after a primary procedure.

Whereas after a first hip or knee replacement we explain to patients they may not feel normal for six months, after a revision surgery, we tell patients they may feel that they are recovering for more than a year. Physical therapy can last twice as long after revision surgery.

Although the exact extent of a revision procedure may not be entirely predictable prior to surgery, the likely options can be anticipated. These options should enable you to discuss with your surgeon the various recovery possibilities and the resources necessary to deal with these possibilities.

Conclusion

A Patient's Perspective: Ron

BY THE MIDDLE OF SUMMER 1996, I was in serious pain, and it was quite clear that my left prosthesis had loosened considerably. We thus planned revision surgery for early September 1996. As I write this it is approximately nine months following my third hip surgery.

And I feel great—the best I have felt in over twenty years. My left hip is beginning to approach my right hip in functioning and is completely pain free. It was never this good following the first surgery on my left hip because the rehabilitation I received (and did on my own) was not as good, and my left leg was considerably weaker than my right leg when the operation on my right leg was done, thus making rehabilitation of the right considerably easier.

This series of events had a serious impact on me psychologically. I now realize in a more concrete way that these implants are not final solutions. Things can go wrong, and when they do it can be quite serious. I am thus a little more consciously aware of my condition than I was three years ago. My approach to life has not changed much, other than not ice skating (yet), but I think more about the implications of having artificial joints than I had previously.

Psychological Impact of Undergoing Revision Surgery

Much more than before, I think about the future, and, for that matter, the present. I wonder how long my present implants will last, how many more operations I will have to endure, and how I will be following them. I have made the choice to maintain an active lifestyle, but that choice is not risk free. I am willing to take the risks for a number of reasons. We still don't know how long these hips will last when a person does not fall on the ice, and maybe they'll last a long time. Why behave like an invalid now, I ask myself, when I will have plenty of time later, and maybe better reason, to act like an invalid? David keeps getting better at what he does, and who knows what developments might be five to ten years away? And I can tolerate the operations. They're no fun—they're pretty awful, in fact—but I (and you) can recover quickly, and with proper care and advice I (and you) can, it appears, come close to recovering fully.

I do have a sense, different from a few years ago, that I am trapped in a deviant physical condition. But it is not much of a burden. It is just an awareness that things are not quite normal. Over the last few years, my wife Julie had a struggle with diabetes, progressing from having no disease to being insulin-dependent in a little over a year. This means that she went from being completely healthy, and thus able to be quite cavalier about eating and drinking habits, to being on an insulin regimen that requires checking blood sugar levels numerous times a day and giving herself shots of insulin. Her whole life was reordered in a blindingly short amount of time, during which she went from being typically unreflective about her health (one of the luxuries of being healthy), to being trapped in a strict regimen that will last the rest of her life.

A Sense of Well-Being and Acceptance

I commented one time to her that I was astounded by how well she was coping with her diabetes (which is not to say that she did not go through a difficult period; she did). Julie told me that it became routine after a while. She could see a somewhat incredulous look in my eye, and she said to me: Do you feel trapped by having to breathe or to eat? When you breathe and eat you provide yourself with necessary nutrients. I basically do the same thing when I give myself insulin. You cope with what you have.

There you have it. You cope with what you have.

Those of us with orthopedic problems have issues peculiar to us, but everyone has issues peculiar to them. We're all trapped in our bodies, with an infinite variety of problems and potential. I have some problems to deal with and think about, but so, too, does everybody else. For me, this was a comforting insight, although it has absolutely no programmatic implications other than this: Don't give up. You must, as I do, live with the risk of failure of these implants. It is now just part of the landscape. Not the most pleasant one, to be sure, but a bearable one. It looks like the surgical techniques are continuing to improve, but you must constantly trade off short- and long-term implications of behavior and aspirations. I have been sobered by this latest series of events, but I remain basically as optimistic and thankful as I have ever been. Indeed, I have now convinced myself that I would have not fallen on the ice had I adequately rehabilitated my left hip the first time around, and I use that as motivation to stick with my conditioning regimen.

Some Final Thoughts
As I have related throughout this book, in all three cases following surgery, things proceeded well during the first months. In each case, however, approximately six months following the surgery, I had a setback. About six months after surgery on my left leg in 1988, I developed a fairly intense pain in my left thigh. Six months after the first surgery on my right hip, the hip stiffened up considerably so that I no longer could flex or extend it very easily. Following the second operation on my left hip, I began experiencing groin and thigh pain, again about six months after surgery. In all three cases, the discomfort was serious, and it persisted for a considerable time. It was serious and durable enough that in each case I went back to David and Vicky with great anxiety that something had gone wrong. The only thing that was ever found was some extra bone growth (ectopic bone) in the muscles surrounding my left hip.

The pain and discomfort were serious enough, and resistant enough to improvement, that I could easily understand how a person might just give up and think that things are not going to get any better. In each case, however, I was able to work through the problems and restore the hip to the condition it was in prior to these acute onsets of discomfort. So the moral of this story is two-fold. First, don't be surprised if you have setbacks, even if a fairly long time has passed since surgery, and even though things have been going fairly well. Second, my experience indicates that these setbacks are temporary, and that you can often work through them. If this happens to you, you need to take it seriously and consult your doctors. Something may actually be wrong. But if your doctor believes everything to be in order, my advice would be to follow through on a sensible rehabilitation regimen. My experience suggests that you will get through this barrier. And once through this last barrier, you should have many years of comfort and freedom of movement from your new joint.

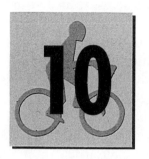

The FUTURE of CARE for ARTHRITIS of the HIP and KNEE

THE PROSPECTS FOR DRAMATIC improvements in all aspects of medical care have probably never been as great as they are now. This is also true for the medical management of hip and knee problems. Over the next few years, advances will vastly increase our understanding of the causes of arthritis of the hip and knee, greatly expand our ability to treat hip and knee ailments—surgically and non-surgically—and significantly alter the way that care for these conditions is financed. In this chapter, you will get a sense of the direction these advances will take so you can manage your own hip and knee care better.

PERHAPS THE SINGLE MOST IMPORTANT development in medical care is the rapidly emerging ability of both patients and physicians to have access to unlimited medical and alternative-medical information. This access will profoundly affect the way all patients, including those with hip and knee problems, receive medical care.

Increased Accessibility of Information

Historically, patients have relied on physicians for information about their medical conditions. Since the 1960s, however, patients have also been able to obtain substantial information in libraries from all types of printed materials and many other sources. In addition, since the early 1990s patients have gained access to an enormous amount of medical information from sources on the internet. The ability of individuals to obtain information via their home computers is profoundly altering the way medical care is being practiced, and it will have an even greater effect in the future.

How to Obtain Information

From your home you can obtain information about the latest and best care from institutions all over the world.

SEEK AS MUCH INFORMATION as possible about your hip or knee problem. As we suggest in earlier chapters, first ask your physician to suggest some articles or programs at institutions that you could consult. Then follow up on materials suggested by those sources. For general information, search sources such as medical books; for more specific and more current information that has been reviewed by professionals, search medical journals; for information about cutting-edge research and programs worldwide, search the internet. But be aware that not all information on the internet is accurate, so be careful how you interpret all of the information available to you.

Most major health care institutions now have sites on the world wide web. These sites often have information about specific medical programs, such as care of the hip or knee. Thus, a good place to start searching for useful medical information is to contact the web sites of well-respected health care providers.

What is exciting about the internet technology is that from your home you can obtain information about the latest and best care from institutions all over the world. Thus, you are no longer constrained to the care provided in your specific location, which, if you live in a relatively remote area, might not be the most current.

If respected medical sources on the web provide information that you believe may be beneficial to you, ask your physician about it. If your physician is unaware of the treatment, suggest that he or she contact the source for further information.

HISTORICALLY, FEW AREAS OF MEDICAL care have been as susceptible to quackery as arthritis care. Numerous remedies for "rheumatism" have been promoted over the years. The potential for quackery, clothed in the jargon of high technology, has never been greater than it is now because of the accessibility of the internet. This potential will increase and be applied to hip and knee conditions with unprecedented fervor and imagination in the coming years.

A Cautionary Note

Unfortunately, in addition to the information from qualified, respected medical care providers available on the internet, a very large amount of information is put on the net by individuals and institutions that are not qualified or accredited to provide medical care. Some of these individuals and institutions may be well-intentioned and interested in providing you with approaches that have helped them deal with their medical problems. Other individuals and institutions may be interested in personally benefiting from giving you advice, regardless of its worth or safety.

If you obtain information from such sources, consult your physician about its usefulness and safety. Because some individuals or institutions that are not qualified or accredited to provide medical advice may have names and titles that sound impressive and legitimate, and may provide real or fabricated credentials and testimonials, consult your physician, a government health department, or a state or national medical or surgical society to confirm the legitimacy of the medical advice being provided.

The freedom of access to medical information available on the internet is making it possible for all individuals to gain substantial control over their medical care. However, this same freedom is making it difficult for society to control the safety and appropriateness of the provided information. In the U.S., we take for granted the existence of laws (such as state licensing of medical doctors) that protect us from unqualified medical care. Those protections don't exist on the internet, so you must be unusually alert when obtaining advice from this source.

Telemedicine for Physicians

TELEMEDICINE, HEALTH CARE PROVIDERS' USE of computer-based telecommunication systems to carry out medical care, presents fantastic potential benefits for all of us. One of the most exciting potentials of telemedicine is the opportunity it allows for all health care providers to communicate among themselves. Thus, a physician in a remote area can gain access over the internet to the latest approaches to the treatment of any condition. Technologies are rapidly emerging that will allow physicians in any part of the world to be directly assisted by medical and surgical specialists at major medical facilities. Thus, as a patient, you should be able to benefit from the latest approaches to the treatment of hip and knee problems, in general, and even to your specific case, no matter where you live.

Ongoing Research into Causes of Osteo- arthritis

INVESTIGATORS AROUND THE WORLD continue to learn more about the cause of osteoarthritis of the hip and knee. Because many factors influence how osteoarthritis of these joints develops, it is unlikely that researchers will find a cure in the next few years. However, it is very likely that they will make substantial progress to influence many of the factors that affect the rate at which the disease progresses in these joints.

For example, as researchers collect more information about the injuries of the knee that increase the risk of developing arthritis, treatment of these injuries will become more effective and the likelihood of developing arthritis from these injuries will decrease. Similarly, researchers likely will determine the mechanisms of certain drugs, such as corticosteroids, which predispose the hip and knee to arthritis, and they will begin to develop methods for blocking the harmful effects of these drug on joints. Finally, researchers will certainly discover many of the genetic factors associated with osteoar-thritis. These discoveries may lead to drugs or procedures that delay or reduce the likelihood of osteoarthritis of the hip and knee.

It is not clear at this time how information obtained from research will be used to reduce the incidence or to slow the progress of osteoarthritis of the hip and knee. Claims undoubt-edly will be made that alterations in diet, ingestion of various vitamins or herbs, and even certain exercise regimens will reduce the likelihood of developing arthritis. Very little infor-mation suggests that these approaches will actually result in an arthritis cure.

Medications

THE NUMBER OF MEDICATIONS AVAILABLE to treat arthritis of the hip and knee will also increase substantially over the next few years. Drugs will be developed to slow the progress of the disease; to treat the signs, such as swelling; and to reduce the symptoms, such as pain and stiffness, of these joints.

Many compounds containing components of normal joint cartilage are now becoming available. These compounds have intuitive appeal, for they seem to make possible the re-placement of the parts of the joint that are being lost as arthri-tis progresses. The popularity of shark cartilage is an example. Preparations of joint fluid components, such as hyaluronic acid, to be taken by mouth or injected, will become available. The ways these compounds work and the impact they have on the progression of arthritis will have to be clarified and the extent of their effectiveness will have to be proven before we can believe such claims. Because osteoarthritis is caused by many factors, it seems unlikely that a single drug that cures and stops arthritis will become available in the near future, despite the headlines of supermarket tabloids.

However, many drugs likely will become available that will treat the signs and symptoms of osteoarthritis more ef-fectively than is currently possible. Researchers are identify-ing many ways that the process of arthritis produces signs and symptoms. For instance, although some of the compounds, such as hyaluronic acid, may not alter the progression of the arthritic process, they may substantially reduce the amount of swelling, stiffness, and pain caused by arthritis. In addition, innovative methods for delivering these compounds, such as skin patches, creams, and self-injectables, are likely to be developed and be useful. Although several promising interventions are currently being developed and tested, at present there are no drugs, vitamins, diets, or other supplements that have proved to change the course of arthritis.

Exercise Programs

SURGEONS AND PHYSICAL THERAPISTS are placing increased emphasis on exercise as a way of controlling the symptoms of arthritis and maintaining function. As the overall beneficial effects of exercise become appreciated, the emphasis on its role in the treatment of arthritis will increase.

The development of exercise programs and equipment specifically for the hip and knee will also increase. A few years ago, individuals with arthritis were routinely advised by their doctors not to perform vigorous exercise. They were specifically warned against leg strengthening exercise, as it was feared that the added stress would accelerate joint deterioration. Swimming was recommended as it was considered the safest and best form of exercise for the arthritic hip and knee because it took weight off these joints. It is now clear that many other activities and exercises more precisely target the issues important to the arthritic hip and knee.

In the past, exercise programs for arthritic hips and knees have benefited from rehabilitation programs initially developed for sports-related injuries to these joints. Because more individuals are participating in sports later in their lives, the number of injuries to these joints is likely to increase. The treatment of these injuries focuses mainly on rehabilitation techniques. The new programs and equipment that will be developed to treat the hip and knee injuries of the senior athlete will undoubtedly be useful in the treatment of arthritis of these joints.

If studies continue to show that exercise reduces the need for more expensive forms of medical care, such as drugs, medical visits, and surgery, then insurance programs are likely to provide increasing incentives for patients with arthritis of the hip and knee to exercise. The day may even come when insurance companies provide patients with incentives to join health clubs! As the demand for exercise as a method of treating arthritis increases, new types of exercise programs and equipment are sure to emerge and be heavily promoted. You will have to be careful in confronting the increasing emphasis on exercise programs for arthritis of the hip and knee, and be sure that the programs you choose are appropriate and safe for you.

New Surgical Techniques and Implants

THE DEVELOPMENT OF NEW SURGICAL techniques to treat arthritis at all stages of the disease is likely to continue at a rapid pace. Evolution of these new techniques will proceed in two directions: improvement of the current procedures, especially joint replacements; and development of new, less invasive procedures.

Total joint replacements are likely to remain the treatment of choice for patients of all ages with advanced arthritis of the hip and knee. Changes in these procedures will be directed toward making the implants more durable, especially for younger, active, or larger patients, and making the procedures safer and more reproducible.

Increasing Implant Durability

SUBSTANTIAL EFFORTS WILL CONTINUE to improve the durability of the polyethylenes used in current designs of total joint replacements. Substantial progress has been made in this area recently, and this progress is likely to continue at a rapid rate. Alternatives to polyethylene as a weight-bearing surface will also be developed and evaluated. The shapes of current implants, particularly total knee implants, will be modified to reduce the wear of the bearing surfaces. The way the parts of the total joint work together may also be modified to increase implant longevity.

Efforts will also continue to improve the durability of the bone cement that is used to hold most hip and knee implants to bone. New bioactive bone cements will be developed that provide initial rigid fixation of the total joint implants and are then replaced by the patient's own bone. Many of these compounds will be genetically engineered, making them completely bio-compatible and safe. Revision of implants inserted using bioactive cements may be easier because more bone will be available in which to place an implant rather than less bone, as is true now. Coatings of implants for use without cement will also be improved to increase the likelihood of secure, long-term fixation. Such coatings are currently being vigorously developed and evaluated. Thus, patients undergoing total joint replacements in the near future will have implants that are likely to last twenty years or more, even if subjected to substantial activity.

It is important, however, if you are contemplating total joint surgery in the near future, to realize that the hip and knee implants and bone cements that are currently available appear to be capable, if inserted correctly, of lasting a very long time, perhaps over twenty years. Even patients who are very active can expect current implants to last that long. Thus, for the majority of patients who currently undergo total joint surgery, it is not necessary or, perhaps, advisable to receive implants made of materials or inserted with materials that do not have a history of many years of use. It takes a decade or two of clinical experience before the durability of a new total joint implant can be assessed. As we have said, the emerging new implants are most appropriate for young, active patients whose life expectancy is substantially greater than the expected longevity of current implants (that is, twenty years).

A GREAT DEAL OF RESEARCH will be done in the next few years to improve the safety of total joint surgery and total joint implants. As more implants are inserted into very elderly patients, the immediate post-operative management of these patients will become increasingly critical. The accurate assessment of pre-operative risk factors in this group of patients will be essential. The likelihood of post-operative complications in very elderly patients will also have to be carefully assessed. It is already clear that the very elderly benefit greatly from a successful total joint procedure. These operations are humane, safe, and cost-effective. Thus, there will be increasing demand for them. Patients of all ages will benefit from the increasing frequency of total joint surgery in the elderly. The specialized techniques developed to ensure that total joint surgery is safe in the very elderly will also ensure that the procedures are safe in younger patients.

Efforts will increase to determine the long-term safety of total joint implants. As we evaluate patients with implants that have been in place for fifteen to twenty years, we will obtain answers to questions that are critical to young patients, such as Ron, who undergo total joint replacement surgery.

Questions being asked include the following: Does the bone around total joint implants remain strong as patients age? Do the wear products of the materials used in total joints, such as metal and plastic, cause adverse systemic side effects as they accumulate? Do these wear products cause cancer? Do they cause genetic abnormalities in the offspring of patients who have had joint replacements? Are some patients more susceptible to systemic effects of wear debris than others? The materials used in total joint replacements, unlike silicone, for example, have been associated with virtually no systemic side effects thus far. However, as the length of time in which these devices have been implanted increases, we will have to be more alert for the emergence of such side effects. Techniques are currently being developed to measure the amounts of wear material in the bodies of patients with total joint implants. Such techniques will be

Making Total Joint Implantation Safer

essential as our experience with these devices, particularly in young people, increases.

Inserting Joint Replacements More Accurately

CONTINUED EFFORTS WILL BE MADE to ensure that total joint implants are inserted accurately and reproducibly. The one factor most influencing the successful function and durability of total joint implants is surgical technique. Remarkable improvements have been made since the 1980s in the techniques used to insert total hip and knee replacements. Total joint replacement surgery is one of the most consistent and reproducible types of surgery performed. Nevertheless, continued improvements in the ways these procedures are performed are sure to occur. Instruments will be developed to increase the accuracy of the procedures.

One of the most exciting innovations in surgery is the use of computer-assisted techniques. These techniques, such as using a robot, are likely to take the accuracy with which joint replacements are performed to a new, higher level. Computer-assisted surgical techniques will also greatly improve the reproducibility with which these procedures are performed. Perhaps the most exciting prospective application of computer-assisted surgical technologies will be their use in the training of surgeons to perform total joint procedures. The day is not far off when surgical simulations, similar to the flight simulations used by airline pilots, will be available. Such simulations will revolutionize the way surgeons are trained and certified.

Less Invasive Procedures

ALTHOUGH VIGOROUS EFFORTS TO IMPROVE total joint surgery will continue as they have since the 1970s, perhaps the area of greatest activity in surgery of the hip and knee will be in the development of new procedures that are less invasive than total joint replacements. Patients have always preferred less invasive procedures. Now, the economic pressures to reduce the costs of medical care are creating additional incentives for their development.

ARTHROSCOPIC SURGERY IS ONE FORM of minimally invasive joint surgery. Although a very useful procedure for the treatment of ligament instabilities and cartilage tears of the knee, its importance in the treatment of arthritic conditions is relatively limited. This may change in the next few years as new technologies expand the potential applications of arthroscopic surgery.

Arthroscopic surgical techniques, or similar minimally invasive procedures, may also be adaptable to certain types of joint replacement, especially of the knee. Techniques are now being developed to integrate the use of computer-assisted surgical technologies and the arthroscope to enable certain types of total knee implants to be accurately implanted. It remains to be seen whether the potential advantages of inserting total knee implants using minimally invasive techniques—that is, faster recovery, less pain, and shorter hospital stay—allows artificial joints to function as well and last as long as total knee implants inserted using current conventional methods.

Arthroscopic Surgery

ANOTHER TECHNOLOGY IS TRANSPLANTED cartilage. It has long been the dream of those taking care of patients with arthritis to be able to grow cartilage on the surface of joints that are degenerating. Many different approaches have been tried with very little success. The biology and bio-mechanical characteristics of weight-bearing joints make successful transplantation and growth of cartilage cells very difficult. Nevertheless, the prospect of being able to reverse the degenerative process by implanting and growing new, healthy cartilage has been so seductive that each new effort has been greeted with great interest and optimism by both the medical profession and the general public. The development of reliable cartilage cell culture techniques and genetic engineering capabilities has heightened the interest in cartilage transplantation.

Many joint conditions, particularly those involving the knee joint, will benefit greatly in the next few years from the research efforts that are currently underway. However, the relevance of this work to the treatment of degenerative

Transplanted Cartilage

arthritis is still not clear. Therefore, it is important for patients, particularly those with knee problems, to understand how relevant cartilage transplantation is to their condition. Cartilage transplantation as it is currently conceived and executed is not an appropriate treatment for a joint with degenerative articular cartilage changes.

The Impact of Medical Costs on Future Hip and Knee Care

ALL OF THESE NEW DEVELOPMENTS, surgical and non-surgical, will be significantly influenced by the U.S. economy and current trends in the management of health care. Medical care systems will no longer pay for new technologies unless they provide equivalent or superior results at lower prices than current technologies. Insurance companies, both public and private, have not been willing to include in their pricing calculations the long-term costs of medical treatment. Thus, for example, though it is well known that the cost of a revision total joint replacement is much greater than the cost of a primary replacement, insurance programs are not currently inclined or organized to pay for more costly primary replacements that might reduce the need for future revision surgery.

The relatively short-term focus of current insurance organizations will have a significant effect on future developments related to care of hip and knee problems. There will be strong financial incentives to use treatment techniques that reduce short-term costs, more or less regardless of the longer term consequences. Thus, surgical procedures on the hip and knee that reduce costs—with less expensive implants, shorter lengths of stay, and less rehabilitation—will be encouraged as long as the relatively short-term results (one to two years) are equivalent to more expensive procedures.

Moreover, unless information emerges that shows convincingly that the surgical treatment of severe arthritis is more cost-effective to society than non-surgical treatment, insurance programs are likely to make access to surgery increasingly difficult. Patients needing joint replacements in the U.S. have not experienced a wait of months or years as have patients in other parts of the world, most notably England and Canada. This situation may change in America for a number of reasons. Insurance companies may, as they already have in many countries, allocate reduced resources to joint replacement procedures, thereby restricting the number that can be done in a given geographic area or at a given hospital. Or the surgical fees for performing these procedures may continue to decrease to a level that discourages orthopedists from performing more than a certain number of procedures per year.

However, an alternative scenario with regard to hip and knee care, including total joint surgery, may emerge. The capitalistic system has shown a remarkable ability to survive and remain economically healthy in the provision of medical care in the U.S. The costs of total joint surgery have dropped dramatically in the last few years with no compromise in the quality of care. Surgeons and hospitals have been creative in their response to increasing cost pressures. They have shown a great desire to provide timely, high-quality joint care to patients. So far, competition among hospitals has reduced the cost of joint replacement care without lowering quality. It is reasonable to worry that continued pressures on costs will begin to compromise the quality of and reduce access to care for hip and knee problems. But health care organizations appear capable of remaining innovative and responsive to patient needs in spite of these significant economic pressures.

Competition among hospitals has reduced the cost of joint replacement care without lowering quality.

THUS, THE FUTURE FOR THE CARE of hip and knee problems appears to be bright. Future care, however, will require more involvement by *you*, the patient, to be successful. As Ron's case illustrates, active patient involvement is the greatest assurance that the quality of hip and knee care will continue to improve, regardless of economic pressures. Your medical outcome, as Ron's experience emphasizes, will only be as good as the amount of effort you put into it.

A Bright Future Ahead

Index

A

Abduction, hip, 19, 20, 21. *See also* Exercise programs; Physical changes, of the hip
Abductor splint, 158
Abnormalities, of joints, 14–15, 21–22
    chromosome, 16
    congenital, 11, 17
    developmental, 91, 92
    genetic, 225
    heterotopic ossification, 158, 163, 177
Acetabular component, 77, 78, 92, 124, 127, 202, 208, 209, 211
    inserting, 124–125
    securing (fixing), 95, 125, 129
Acetabulum (cup), 69, 77, 78, 124, 125, 127
Acetaminophen (active ingredient in Tylenol), 45, 48, 49, 64, 107, 143. *See also* Analgesics
Activities, daily, 31–39
    carrying things, 38
    chairs, getting in and out of, 30, 31, 37, 158
    climbing stairs, 6, 18, **25**, 31, 37, 38, **191**
    dressing, 31, 33–34, **35–36**, 158
    personal hygiene, 31–33, 158
    sitting, 14, **25**, 30, 37, 38, 158, **191**
    using the bathroom, 31, 32–33
    vehicles, getting in and out of, **24**, **25**, 30, 31, 37, 38, **58**, 158
    walking, 14, 18, 24, 37, 41, **191**
    working, 38–39
Acupuncture, 52. *See also* Alternative treatments and medicines
Adaptive equipment (assistive devices), 31–38, 74, 169, 212
    availability of, 31, 36
    for the bathroom, 32–33, 146, 158
        bath bench, 32, 33, 146
        elevated toilet seat, 32, 33, 146, 158
        handrails, 32–33
        long-handled sponge, 32
    for dressing, 33–36, 146, 158
        dressing sticks, 34, 35
        extended handle shoe horns, 34, 35
        reachers, 34, 35, 146, 158
        sock donners, 34, 34, 158
    purchase of, 36–37
    shoe lift, 165–166
    for walking, 37

Adduction, hip, 21
Advancements, in medical treatment. *See* Medical advancements
Aerobic exercise, 183, **191**, **192**. *See also* Exercise
    benefits of, 29, 171, 172
    program, 178–179, 190
Aging. *See* Elderly persons
Allen, Ron, ii, 3, 4–10, **23–25**, **31**, **35**, **40**, **44**, **49–51**, **57**, **58–59**, **75–80**, 77–78, **90**, 92, 96, 97, 116, **118–119**, **121**, **123**, **143**, **150**, **157**, **176–177**, **178–179**, **190–194**, **198–199**, **200**, 201, **202–203**, 204–208, **212–215**, 225, 229
Alternative treatments and medicines, 51–54. *See also* Drug therapy; Surgery; Therapy; Treatment
    acupuncture, 52
    biofeedback, 51
    chiropractic manipulation, 52
    commonly asked-about, 52
    massage, 51
    meditation, 51
    unproven medications, 53–54
American Academy of Orthopaedic Surgery, 81, 83
Analgesia, 46, 120
Analgesic(s), 47–48, 114. *See also* Drug therapy; Medication(s)
    acetaminophen, 45, 48
    dosage, 47
    effectiveness, 47
    narcotic derivatives, 48, 64, 143, 155, 168
    post-surgical use of, 120, 143
    pumps, 143
    side effects, 47, 48
Anesthesia/anesthetic, **118–119**, 119–121, 130
    administering of, 116, 119–121, 123
    as cause of constipation, 154
    combined, 120–121, **121**
    fear of, 72, **118**, 119
    general, 67, 71, 117, 119, 120, **121**
    local, 67, 119, 210
    regional (epidural or spinal), 67, 71, 117, 119–120, **121**
Anesthesiologist, 83, 112, 116, 117, **121**
Ankylosing spondylitis (DISH Syndrome), 17, 163
Anterior cruciate ligament (meniscus), 66–67, 68, 69. *See also* Ligaments